POWER
VS.
FORCE

Please visit:

Hay House USA: www.hayhouse.com®
Hay House Australia: www.hayhouse.com.au
Hay House UK: www.hayhouse.co.uk
Hay House India: www.hayhouse.co.in

POWER
vs.
FORCE

The Hidden Determinants
of Human Behavior

David R. Hawkins, M.D., Ph.D.

Author's Official Authoritative Edition

HAY HOUSE, INC.
Carlsbad, California • New York City
London • Sydney • New Delhi

Published in the United States by: Hay House, Inc.: www.hayhouse.com®
Published in Australia by: Hay House Australia Pty. Ltd.: www.hayhouse.com.au
Published in the United Kingdom by: Hay House UK, Ltd.: www.hayhouse.co.uk
Published in India by: Hay House Publishers India: www.hayhouse.co.in

Previously published by Veritas Publishing (ISBN 978-0964326-11-8)
1st Hay House printing, February 2002

Library of Congress Control Number: 2013945703

Tradepaper ISBN: 978-1-4019-4507-7

31 30 29 28 27 26 25
1st Hay House printing, author's official authoritative edition,
December, 2013

Printed in the United States of America

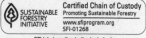

Certified Chain of Custody
SUSTAINABLE   Promoting Sustainable Forestry
FORESTRY
INITIATIVE   www.sfiprogram.org
              SFI-01268

SFI label applies to the text stock

The skillful are not obvious
They appear to be simple-minded
Those who know this know the patterns
of the Absolute
To know the patterns is the Subtle Power
The Subtle Power moves all things and has no name

———◆———

DEDICATION

Gloria in Excelsis Deo!

TABLE OF CONTENTS

IMAGINE—WHAT if you had access to a simple yes-or-no (Y/N) answer to any question you wished to ask. A demonstrably true answer. Any question, phrased as a statement.

Think about it.

There's the obvious: "Jane is seeing another guy." (Y/N). "Johnny is telling the truth about school." (Y/N). But it's only a short step to: "This is a safe investment." (Y/N). "This career is worthy of my pursuit." (Y/N).

What if everyone had such access?

Staggering implications suggest themselves immediately. Think again.

What would happen to our ponderous and all-too-often flawed judicial system if there were a clear, confirmable answer to the proposition, "John Doe is guilty as charged." (Y/N)?

What would happen to politics as we know it if all of us could ask the question, "Candidate X honestly intends to fulfill this campaign promise." (Y/N)—and all of us got the same answer?

And what would happen to advertising, period?

You get the idea. But the idea gets bigger, fast. What happens to nationalism ("Nation X is in fact dedicated to the overthrow of Democracy.")? To government ("This bill does in fact protect the rights of citizens.")?

What happens to "The check is in the mail"?

If, as has been said, man learned to lie an hour after he learned to talk, then a phenomenon such as the one we're discussing would be the genesis of the most fundamental change in human knowledge since the beginning of society; the transformations it would wreak—in fields from communications to ethics, in our most basic concepts, in every detail of daily existence—would be so profound that it is difficult to even conceive what life would be like in a subsequent new era of truth. The world as we know it would be irrevocably changed, right down to its very roots.

—

kinesiology: -n. The study of muscles and their movements, esp. as applied to physical conditioning. [Gk. Kinesis, movement (kinein, to move) + -logy.][1]

The study of kinesiology first received scientific attention in the second half of the last century through the work of Dr. George Goodheart, who pioneered the specialty he called *applied kinesiology* after finding that benign physical stimuli—for instance, beneficial nutritional supplements—would increase the strength of certain indicator muscles, whereas inimical stimuli would cause those muscles to suddenly weaken.[2] The implication was that at a level far below conceptual consciousness, the body "knew," and through muscle testing was able to signal, what was good and bad for it. The classic example, cited later in this work, is a universally observed weakening of indicator muscles in the presence of a chemical sweetener; the same muscles strengthen in the presence of a healthful, natural supplement.

In the late 1970s, Dr. John Diamond refined this specialty into a new discipline he called *behavioral kinesiology*. Dr. Diamond's startling discovery was that indicator muscles would strengthen or weaken in the presence of positive or negative emotional and intellectual stimuli, as well as physical stimuli.[3] A smile will make you test strong, while the statement, "I hate you," will make you test weak.

Before we go any further, let us explain in detail exactly how one "tests," especially as the reader will certainly wish to try this himself. Here is Dr. Diamond's outline, from his 1979 book, *Your Body Doesn't Lie*, of the procedure adapted by him from the classic description in H. O. Kendall's *Muscles: Testing and Function* (Baltimore: Williams & Wilkins, 2nd ed., 1971).

It takes two people to perform a kinesiological test. Choose a friend or a family member for testing. We'll call him or her your subject.

1. Have the subject stand erect, right arm relaxed at his side, left arm held out parallel to the floor, elbow straight. (You may use the other arm if you wish.)
2. Face your subject and place your left hand on his right shoulder to steady him. Then place your right hand on the subject's extended left arm just above the wrist.
3. Tell the subject you are going to try to push his arm down as he resists with all his strength.
4. Now push down on his arm fairly quickly, firmly, and evenly. The idea is to push just hard enough to test the spring and bounce in the arm, but not so hard that the muscle becomes fatigued. It is not a question of who is stronger, but of whether the muscle can "lock" the shoulder joint against the push.

Assuming there is no physical problem with the muscle and the subject is in a normal, relaxed state of mind, receiving no extraneous stimuli (for this reason it is important that the tester not smile or otherwise interact with the subject), the muscle will "test strong"—the arm will remain locked. If the test is repeated in the presence of a negative stimulus (for instance, artificial sweetener), "although you are pushing down no harder than before, the muscle will not be able to resist the pressure and the subject's arm will fall to his side."[4]

A striking aspect of Diamond's research was the uniformity of response among his subjects. Diamond's results were predictable, repeatable, and universal. This was so even where no rational link existed between stimulus and response. For totally undetermined reasons, certain abstract symbols caused all subjects to test weak; others, the opposite. Some results were perplexing: certain pictures, with no overtly positive or negative content would cause all subjects to test weak, while other "neutral" pictures caused all subjects to test strong. And some results were food for considerable surmise: Whereas virtually all classical music and most pop music (including "classic" rock and roll) caused a universally strong response, the "hard" or "metal" rock that first gained popularity in the late 1970s produced a universally weak response.

There was one other phenomenon that Diamond noted in passing, though devoting no deeper analysis to its extraordinary implications. Subjects listening to tapes of known deceits—Lyndon Johnson perpetrating the Tonkin Gulf hoax, Edward Kennedy stonewalling the Chappaquiddick incident—universally tested weak. While listening to recordings of demonstrable, true statements, they universally tested strong.[5] This was the starting point of the work of the author of this volume, the well-known psychiatrist and physician, David R. Hawkins. In 1975, Dr. Hawkins began research on the kinesiologic response to truth and falsehood.

It had been established that test subjects did not need any conscious acquaintance with the substance (or issue) being tested. In double-blind studies—and in mass demonstrations involving entire lecture audiences—subjects universally tested weak in response to unmarked envelopes containing artificial sweetener, and strong to identical placebo envelopes. The same naïve response appeared in testing intellectual values.

What seems to be at work is a form of communal consciousness, *spiritus mundi*, or as Hawkins calls it, following Jung, a "database of consciousness." The phenomenon seen so commonly in other social animals—whereby a fish swimming at one edge of a school will turn instantaneously when its fellows a quarter mile away flee a predator—pertains in some subconscious way to our species also. There are simply too many documented instances of individuals having intimate acquaintance with information experienced firsthand by remote strangers for us to deny that there are forms of shared knowledge other than those achieved by rational consciousness. Or perhaps, more simply, the same spark of inner sub-rational wisdom that can discriminate healthy from unhealthy can discriminate true from false.

One highly suggestive element of this phenomenon is the binary nature of the response. Hawkins found that questions must be phrased so that the answer is very clearly yes or no, like a nerve synapse that is on or off; like the most basic cellular forms of "knowledge"; like so much of what our cutting-edge physicists tell us is the essential nature of universal energy. Is the human brain, at some primal level, a wondrous computer linked with a universal energy field that knows far more than it knows it knows?

Be that as it may. As Dr. Hawkins's research continued, his most fertile discovery was a means of calibrating a scale of relative truth by which intellectual positions, statements, or ideologies could be rated on a range of 1 to 1,000. One can say, "This item (book, philosophy, teacher) calibrates at 200 (Y/N), at 250 (Y/N)," and so on, until the point of common weak response determines the calibration. The enormous implication of these calibrations was that for the first time in human history, ideological validity could be appraised as an innate quality in any subject.

Through twenty years of similar calibrations, Hawkins was able to analyze the full spectrum of the levels of human consciousness, developing a fascinating map of the geography of man's experience. This "anatomy of consciousness" produces a profile of the entire human condition, allowing a comprehensive analysis of the emotional and spiritual development of individuals, societies, and the race in general. So profound and far-reaching a view provides not only a new understanding of man's journey in the universe, but also a guide to all of us as to where we and our neighbors are on the ladder of spiritual enlightenment, and on our own personal journeys to become who we could be.

In this volume, Dr. Hawkins brings these fruits of decades of research and insight into the penetrating illumination of revolutionary discoveries in advanced particle physics and nonlinear dynamics. For the first time in our Western intellectual record, he shows that the cold light of science is confirming what mystics and saints have always said about the self, God, and the very nature of reality] This vision of being, essence, and divinity presents a picture of man's relation to the universe that is unique in its capacity to satisfy both soul and reason. There is a rich intellectual and spiritual harvest here, much that you can take, and much more that you can give yourself.

Turn the page. The future starts now.

E. Whalen, Editor
Bard Press
Arizona, 1995

ORIGINAL PREFACE

To explain that which is "simple" can be difficult indeed. Much of this book is devoted to the process of making the simple obvious. If we can understand even one simple thing in depth, we will have greatly expanded our capacity for comprehending the nature of the universe and of life itself.

Kinesiology is now a well-established science, based on testing of an all-or-none muscle response to stimuli. A positive stimulus provokes a strong muscle response; a negative stimulus results in a demonstrable weakening of the test muscle. Clinical kinesiologic muscle testing has found widespread verification over the last twenty-five years. Goodheart's original research on the subject was given wider application by Dr. John Diamond, whose books brought the subject to the public. Diamond determined that this positive or negative response occurs with stimuli both physical and mental.

The research reflected in this volume has taken Dr. Diamond's technique several steps further, through the discovery that this kinesiologic response reflects the capacity of the human organism to differentiate not only positive from negative stimuli, but also anabolic (life-enhancing) from catabolic (life-consuming), and, most dramatically, true from false.

The test itself is simple, rapid, and relatively foolproof. A positive muscle reaction occurs in response to a statement that is objectively true; a negative response occurs if the test subject is presented with a false statement. This phenomenon occurs independently of the test subject's own opinion or knowledge of the topic, and the response has proven cross-culturally valid in many populations and consistent through time. The test results thus fulfill the scientific requirement of replication and, therefore, reliable verification by other investigators. This technique provides, for the first time in human history, an objective basis for distinguishing truth from falsehood, which is totally verifiable across time with randomly selected, naïve test subjects.

Moreover, we found that this testable phenomenon can be used to calibrate human levels of consciousness so that an arbitrary logarithmic scale of whole numbers emerges, stratifying the relative power of levels of consciousness in all areas of human experience. Exhaustive investigation has resulted in a calibrated scale of consciousness, in which the log of whole numbers from 1 to 1,000 calibrates the degree of power of all possible levels of human awareness.

The millions of calibrations that confirmed this discovery further disclosed a stratification of levels of power in human affairs, revealing a remarkable distinction between power and force and their respective qualities. This, in turn, led to a comprehensive reinterpretation of human behavior in order to identify the invisible energy fields that control it. The calibrated scale was found to coincide with sublevels of the hierarchy of the *perennial philosophy*; correlations with emotional and intellectual phenomena in sociology, clinical psychology, psychoanalysis, and traditional spirituality immediately suggested themselves.

The calibrated scale has been examined here in light of current discoveries in advanced theoretical physics and the nonlinear dynamics of *chaos theory*. Calibrated levels, we suggest, represent powerful attractor Fields within the domain of consciousness

INVISIBLE ENERGY FIELDS CONTROLLING HUMAN BEHAVIOR

itself, which dominate human existence and therefore define content, meaning, and value, and serve as organizing energies for widespread patterns of human behavior.

This stratification of attractor Fields, according to corresponding levels of consciousness, provides a new paradigm for recontextualizing the human experience throughout all time. Practically, by accessing data to which there has heretofore been no avenue of approach, our method promises both great value in researching history and enormous possible benefit for man's future. In attempting to emphasize the value of this technique as a research tool, examples have been given of its potential uses in a wide range of human activities: speculatively, in art, history, commerce, politics, medicine, sociology, and the natural sciences; pragmatically, in marketing, advertising, research and development; and empirically, in psychological, philosophic, and spiritual-religious inquiry. Specific applications have been suggested in such diverse fields as criminology, intelligence, addictionology, and the whole field of self-improvement.

But further uses and extrapolations of the research method detailed herein have been barely hinted at. Although the results described here are the product of twenty years of investigation and millions of calibrations on thousands of subjects by teams of investigators, this book represents only a beginning exploration of the method's potential to enhance our knowledge in all of the arts and sciences. Perhaps most important is its promise as an aid in spiritual growth and maturation to the most advanced levels of consciousness, even enlightenment itself.

By use of the kinesiologic testing procedure described herein, unlimited information about any subject, past or present, is universally available. But the realization that everything is knowable about anything or anyone, anywhere, at any point in time, creates at first a paradigm shock. This reaction arises, generally, from realization of the nonlocality, impersonality and universality of consciousness itself; and, specifically, from the realization of the observability of one's own thoughts and motivations, and their transparency across time. That one's every thought and action leave an indelible trace forever in the universe can be an unsettling thought.

As in the case of the discovery of radio waves or x-rays, a sudden expansion of our awareness of the workings of the universe not only allows but demands a recontextualization of our worldview. Implications of new knowledge require a reworking of old ideas to form a larger context. Though it may occasion some intellectual stress, such scientific recontextualization of human behavior can expose the basic structures that underlie personal and social problems, thereby revealing their potential solutions.

Because this subject matter is, in fact, extraordinarily simple, it is difficult to present in a world enamored of complexity. Despite our mistrust of simplification, we may see two general classes of people in the world: believers and nonbelievers. To the nonbelievers, everything is false until proven true; to the believers, everything said in good faith is probably true unless it is proven false. The pessimistic position of cynical skepticism stems from fear. The more optimistic manner of accepting information arises from self-confidence. Either style works and each has its pros and cons. I have been faced, therefore, with the problem of presenting the data in a manner that will satisfy both approaches.

This book is, therefore, oxymoronic in style, written to facilitate both so-called left- and right-brain comprehension. In actuality, we know things by a holistic pattern-recognition. The easiest way to grasp an entirely new concept is simply by familiarity. This kind of understanding is encouraged by a style of writing characterized as "closure." Instead of using only sparse adjectives or examples to express thoughts, they are instead run out and completed by use of repetition. The concept is then "done," and the mind is left at ease. Such an approach is also desirable because the mind that reads Chapter 3 will not be the same as the mind that reads Chapter 1.

For that matter, the idea of having to start from Chapter 1 and read progressively to the end is merely a fixed left-brain concept. This is the pedestrian path of Newtonian physics, based on a limited and limiting view of the world in which all events supposedly happen in an A→B→C sequence. This form of myopia arises from an outdated paradigm of reality. Our wider and far more comprehensive view draws not only upon the essence of the most advanced physics, mathematics, and nonlinear theory, but also upon intuitions that can be experientially validated by anyone.

In general, the challenge in presenting this material lies in the paradox of comprehending nonlinear concepts in a linear, sentence-by-sentence structure. The fields of science from which the data emerged are of themselves complex and difficult enough: advanced theoretical physics and the mathematics thereof; nonlinear dynamics; chaos theory and its mathematics; advanced behavioral kinesiology; neurobiology; turbulence theory; as well as the philosophic considerations of epistemology and ontology. Beyond this, it was necessary to address the nature of human consciousness itself, an uncharted area at the perimeter of which the sciences have all drawn back. To conclusively comprehend such subjects from a purely intellectual viewpoint would be a staggering enterprise, requiring a lifetime of study. Instead of essaying so formidable a task, I have tried to extract the essence of each subject and work only with these essences.

Even a rudimentary attempt to explain the workings of the testing technique fundamental to this book, which seems initially to transcend known laws of the universe, inevitably leads us into the intellectual territories of advanced theoretical physics, nonlinear dynamics, and chaos theory. I have therefore attempted, as much as possible, to present these subjects in nontechnical terms. There is no need to worry that some erudite intellectual capacity is required to digest this material. It is not; we will circle around the same concepts over and over until they are obvious. Each time we return to comment on an example, greater comprehension will occur. This kind of learning is like surveying new terrain in an airplane: on the first pass, it all looks unfamiliar; the second time around, we spot some points of reference; the third time, it starts to make sense, and we finally gain familiarity through simple exposure. The inborn pattern-recognition mechanism of the mind takes care of the rest.

———

To quell my own fear that perhaps, despite my best efforts, the reader might not get the essential message of this study, I will spell it out in advance: the individual human mind is like a computer terminal connected to a giant database. The database is human consciousness itself, of which our own consciousness is merely an individual expression, but with its roots in the common consciousness of all mankind. This database is the realm of genius; because to be human is to participate in the database, everyone, by virtue of their birth, has access to genius. The unlimited information contained in the database has now been shown to be readily available to anyone in a few seconds, at any time and in any place. This is indeed an astonishing discovery, bearing the power to change lives, both individually and collectively, to a degree never yet anticipated.

The database transcends time, space, and all limitations of individual consciousness. This distinguishes it as a unique tool for future research, and opens as yet undreamed-of areas for possible investigation. It holds forth the prospect of the establishment of an objective basis for human values, behaviors, and belief systems. The information obtained by this method reveals a new context for understanding human behavior and a new paradigm for validating objective truth. Because the technique itself can be used by integrous people, anywhere, at any time, it has the capacity to initiate a new era of human experience based on observable and verifiable truth.

We have at our fingertips a means of accurately distinguishing truth from falsehood, workable from unworkable, benevolent from malign. We can illuminate the hidden forces, hitherto overlooked, that determine human behavior. We have at our disposal a means of finding answers to previously unresolved personal and social problems. Falsehood need no longer hold sway over our lives.

(Subsequent research, following the original 1995 publication of this book, indicates that only people who themselves calibrate 200 or over are able to obtain accurate test results. See Chapter Two and Appendix C for further details.)

Though the subject matter has proven easy to teach in lecture or videotape, the problem has been to work it into readable form. The proofs can be complex. The demonstrations, however, are ultra-simple. Children get it right away and follow with delight. There is nothing here that is surprising to them. They have always known that they were connected to the database; we adults have merely forgotten it. The inherent genius of children is close to the surface, which is why it was children who saw that the emperor was not wearing any clothes. Genius is like that.

This book will have been successful if by the end of it you exclaim, "I always knew that!" What is contained herein is only a reflection of that which you already know, but do not know that you know. All that I have hoped to do here is to connect the dots to let the hidden picture emerge.

This book makes a huge promise, perhaps the biggest promise that has ever been made to you. It can provide you the means by which you may detect if you are being misled. (Therefore, you never need to read a book or buy into any major teaching again without testing it first—it is too dangerous and too costly.) The level of truth of this work itself has been calibrated at 850 (see Appendix A), which is unusually high for this time in our culture. I pray that this is already a partial fulfillment of the promise.

My hope as author has been that this work might undo the very sources of pain, suffering, and failure, and assist the evolution of human consciousness in each of us to rise to the level of joy that should be the essence of man's experience.

—

The work presented by this book began in January, 1965, and was finally finished in June, 1994. Much of the material was originally developed in the course of work on a doctoral dissertation. The findings reported in the study were independently derived by the use of the research tool elucidated herein, the kinesiologic response. The work evolved spontaneously, without reference to outside sources of information; correlation with the work of others was incorporated at a later date to provide an intellectual frame of reference. Much of the work in this study has now been corroborated by worldwide research presented in independent studies, such as the first major conference on consciousness, "Toward a Scientific Basis for Consciousness," held at the University of Arizona Health Sciences Center, Tuscon, Arizona, in April of 1994.[1]

Our research teams used the testing method described in the book to calibrate the levels of truth of every chapter, paragraph, and sentence. (For instance, testing revealed an error in a list of celebrities who had destroyed themselves as a consequence of their fame. When we checked each word, the name "John Lennon" was found to be in error: in fact, he was shot by an assassin. When his name was deleted, the level of truth of the sentence, and therefore the paragraph and the page, rose to match that of the rest of the chapter.)

Preliminary versions of the book were circulated among selected readers, from rank-and-file healthcare workers to heads of state such as Mikhail Gorbachev and Nobel Prize winners; some comments appear on the back cover. Each person's response to the presentation of the subject has been unique. (One interesting fact observed was that the scores of tested individuals increased after encountering the material; it appears that mere exposure to the data "raised" the subjects' level of consciousness.) Because the implications and practical applications of the work are so varied, and any aspect of the material can be expanded and focused to suit the interests of a given audience, portions of it have lent themselves clinically to presentations for various special-interest groups.

A segment of the material was presented by the author in the keynote speech at the First National Conference on Consciousness and Addictions in San Mateo, California, in 1985[2] and a summation was published in the Proceedings of that conference by the Brookridge Institute (*Beyond Addictions, Beyond Boundaries*, edited by Shirley Burton and Leo Kiley, 1986).[3] An expanded version was given in a four-hour videotaped lecture on Consciousness and Addictions at the Second National Conference on Consciousness and Addictions in San Francisco in 1986.[4]

Other parts of the material appeared in a set of

videos published in the 1980s called the "Archival Office Visit Series": Stress; Health; Illness and Self-Healing; Handling Major Crises; Depression; Alcoholism; Spiritual First Aid; The Aging Process; The Map of Consciousness; Death and Dying; Pain and Suffering; Losing Weight; Worry, Fear and Anxiety; Drug Addiction and Alcoholism; and Sexuality.[5]

Some of this material was presented during three-hour weekly lectures given at an alcohol and drug rehabilitation center over a five-year period (1984-1988).

This is the first time the anatomy of consciousness itself has been delineated in pure form in its entirety, without attenuation to the interests of a specific, special-interest audience.

David R. Hawkins, M.D., Ph.D.
The Institute for Spiritual Research
Sedona, Arizona, 1995

NEW FOREWORD

This Revised Edition is vital for several reasons.

In 2006, Dr. Hawkins read the entire book for an audio recording so that listeners would receive not only the book's information but also the "carrier wave" of its context and aura. While reading the book aloud, Dr. Hawkins made spontaneous oral revisions to the text. The Revised Edition incorporates all of those changes.

Most of the revisions are subtle, as in word changes. For instance, in the audio recording, he uses the word "negative" instead of "evil" in some places, the word "source" instead of "cause," etc. A few revisions are substantial, as in a thorough explanation of the muscle-testing method and its use in consciousness research. As Dr. Hawkins worked with this technique over the years, methodological nuances were discovered and integrated.

The Revised Edition also addresses the fact that the calibration of a subject may change over time. In cases where there was a difference between the calibration in the original *Power vs. Force* and a later publication, the Revised Edition includes the later calibration in parentheses. For instance, Chapter 23 on "The Search for Truth" gives the original 1995 calibrations of various religious groups, followed by the calibrations from the later book *Truth vs. Falsehood* (2005) in parentheses. The calibrations of religious groups change over time consequent to changes in their policies. The calibration of a scripture or writing varies according to the particular edition or translation. The calibration of an individual may vary depending on what is held in mind (i.e., their contribution to society, a particular book they wrote, their intention in a specific endeavor, etc.) Moreover, when a subject is calibrated multiple times, this re-addressing may contribute to a change in calibration.

The author's dedication is to be truthful, accurate, and precise. As he explains in the book, *the law of sensitive dependence on initial conditions* means that a slight variation over time can produce a major change in outcome, "much as a ship whose bearing is one degree off compass will eventually find itself hundreds of miles off course." In the Revised Edition, therefore, the effort is made to communicate the "initial conditions" in their most pristine and precise wording.

———

The publication of the Revised Edition of *Power vs. Force* is occurring simultaneously with the author's retirement from public teaching. We have the propitious opportunity, therefore, to review the impact of the book since its original publication over fifteen years ago.

This book brings humanity to its most compelling conjunction thus far between the linear world of logic, reason, and science, and the nonlinear realities of love, joy, beauty, self-transcendence, *unio mystica* and Enlightenment.

Dr. David R. Hawkins is a world-renowned author, psychiatrist, clinician, spiritual teacher, and researcher of consciousness. His unique work effulges from a wellspring of universal compassion and is dedicated to the alleviation of suffering throughout the world and all realms.

By giving confirmation of spiritual Reality as the essence of human life, and Divinity as the source of consciousness, the work reveals every aspect of human experience to be an expression of, and a pathway to, the Ultimate.

In the 1970s, as a physician, he pioneered several integrated approaches in the treatment of severely disturbed psychiatric patients. If Mother Teresa worked with the "poorest of the poor," Dr. Hawkins worked with the "sickest of the sick." His treatments addressed the whole person through physical, mental, and spiritual levels of healing and betterment. In 1973, he co-authored the landmark book, *Orthomolecular Psychiatry*, with Nobel Laureate chemist Linus Pauling, initiating a new field within psychiatry.

In the 1980s, his work changed the face of addiction by putting it into the larger context of the science of consciousness. Alcoholism and addiction affect millions of people; therefore, to light the path out of that despairing place is a tremendous gift to humankind. Dr. Hawkins' work verified that the states of bliss and love sought by the addict and alcoholic could be found within, through interior endeavor and surrender.

> *What the addict is seeking is not to be ashamed of. The whole spiritual world wants to reach that blissful state of consciousness.*
>
> *Change your technique, not your aspiration. The state doesn't have to be sought; it is always within us.*

In the 1990s, his life took an unanticipated turn.

Responsive to friends and loved ones who saw the importance of this book for the world, he self-published *Power vs. Force: Anatomy of Consciousness* in 1995. He was reluctant to use his personal name as the author; experientially, it was written by a source greater than the personal self.

Power vs. Force has been translated into twenty-five languages and has likely sold over a million copies. Ten more books have followed, with hundreds of lectures, radio interviews, and the establishment of Hawkins Study Groups in most major cities around the world, from Seoul to Cape Town to Los Angeles.

———

This book, *Power vs. Force*, transmits a major breakthrough for the human psyche, delineating dimensions of consciousness heretofore known only to the "mystics" of history. Such beings, gifted with a direct realization of Reality (by whatever name), have always confirmed the central importance of the "unseen."

> *The outer work can never be small*
> *if the inner work is great.*
> *And the outer work can never be great*
> *if the inner work is small.*

~ *Meister Eckhart, 14th-century Christian mystic*

They have pointed us, as Meister Eckhart did, to realize our "inner greatness," because everything in the visible world issues from the inner planes. As Dr. Hawkins writes in the opening page of *Power vs. Force*:

The skillful are not obvious
They appear to be simple-minded
Those who know this know the patterns
of the Absolute
To know the patterns is the Subtle Power
The Subtle Power moves all things and
has no name.

For possibly the first time in human history, Dr. Hawkins has given us a body of work that verifies this "mystic truth" through the finest advances of human science, psychology, and philosophy.

A trademark of Hawkins' research is the now well-known "Map of Consciousness" presented in this book. "The Map of Consciousness" confirms that the classical "stages" of human inner evolution found in the world's sacred literature are actual, measurable "attractor patterns" and "energy fields." These levels had been suggested by philosophers, saints, sages, and mystics throughout the centuries; yet there had never been a scientific framework by which to understand them and thereby progress to ultimate freedom. The "Map of Consciousness" is free of dogma and clinically sophisticated in its depiction of the emotional process, view of God, view of self, and view of life true to each level of consciousness.

Power vs. Force presents a logically compelling anatomy of consciousness that lays out the arch of human spiritual evolution from its lowest expression (shame) to its highest (Enlightenment). It illumines the oneness of all creation by revealing the energy essence of everything that exists—human and non-human, seen and unseen. All of life is revealed to be a pulsating symphony of interplaying energies: "The mutual dependence and interpenetration of all things is observable as one leaves duality. Oneness is central to all of the major religions and spiritual systems as the ultimate reality underlying and within all forms."

This book provides the pragmatic and clinical explanation for certain core principles held to be true across cultures: love is more powerful than hatred; truth sets us free; forgiveness liberates both sides; unconditional love heals; courage empowers; and the essence of Divinity/Reality is peace.

While such truths have long been intuitively known in the collective human spirit and confirmed by the rare mystics who directly experienced them, we now have a readily accessible and scientifically contextualized chart that points the way to human freedom.

The levels of consciousness ("energy fields") are calibrated according to their measurable effect. With each progressive rise in the level of consciousness, the "frequency" or "vibration" of energy increases. Thus, higher consciousness radiates a beneficial and healing effect on the world, verifiable in the human muscle response, which stays strong in the presence of love and truth. In contrast, non-true or negative energy fields induce a weak muscle response. That which weakens life energy is to be avoided: shame, guilt, confusion, fear, hatred, pride, hopelessness, and falsehood. That which uplifts life is to be realized: truth, courage, acceptance, reason, love, beauty, joy, and peace.

This discovery of the difference between "power" and "force" has influenced many fields of human endeavor: business, advertising, education, psychology, medicine, law, and international relations. Experts in each field have implemented the mechanisms of success and genius outlined in this book to great effect.

Beyond the light it sheds on ordinary human pursuits of livelihood, health, art, sports, relationships, and politics, *Power vs. Force* constitutes one of the first modern demarcations of the highest levels of human consciousness (Self-Realization, the Void, Nothingness vs. Allness, Full Enlightenment) and their differential phenomena.

The autobiographical essay at the end of this book substantiates the advanced consciousness of its author. It is not necessary that readers value this aspect of the author's life in order to benefit from the book; yet, for scholars, theologians, and seekers who understand the rarity of this state of awareness, this recognition can be profoundly catalytic.

Dr. Hawkins describes the gradations of Enlightenment with a level of clarity that indicates the experiential realization of them. We cannot, after all, draw a map to a place we have not been. In-depth interviews confirm the presence of a very advanced state of consciousness, with all the classic hallmarks: pristine awareness of Ultimate Reality, compassion for all beings, tireless dedication to alleviate suffering, precision and elegance in every word and movement, freedom of being, spontaneity, radiant joy, humor, oneness with all of existence, and a depth of surrender to Reality that is unimaginable to the average person.

As with many great pioneers of the human spirit, the work for which Dr. Hawkins is now renowned began in the depths of his own consciousness. In later books such as *The Eye of the I*, *I: Reality and Subjectivity*, *Discovery of the Presence of God*, and

Transcending the Levels of Consciousness, he explains the highest levels of consciousness in language that is "realized" and inspirational to all walks of life — religious and non-religious, all races, all ages, all nationalities, all personal backgrounds.

The gift of this work to human evolvement is beyond what can be said about it.

Without a map in hand, the treasure cannot be found. This pathway is open to all who choose it. We all have different starting points, yet each of us guides the rudder of our future by our own hands. Substantial progress is made, Dr. Hawkins suggests, by practicing any true principle, such as: "Be kind and forgiving to everything and everyone, including yourself, at all times without exception."

In 2003, the students of his work requested that Dr. Hawkins give a name to the body of teachings. "Devotional Nonduality" was the response, harmonizing what has historically been viewed as opposites in the inner journey: the heart and the mind. The teachings of Devotional Nonduality emphasize the core truths of the world's great spiritual traditions: kindness and compassion to everything and everyone (including oneself), humility, forgiveness, simplicity, lovingness as a way of being, reverence for all of life, devotion to Truth, and surrender to God. It is a direct path to Enlightenment in which each internal progression of love and integrity uplifts the whole of existence:"We change the world not by what we say or do but as a consequence of what we have become."

Similar to other advanced teachers (Mother Teresa, Ramana Maharshi), seekers come from far-flung places to be in his presence, stating that the "aura" or

DEVOTIONAL NON-DUALITY — EMPHASIZE KINDNESS & COMPASSION, HUMILITY, FORGIVENESS, SIMPLICITY — REVERENCE FOR ALL LIFE, DEVOTION TO TRUTH, SURRENDER TO GOD.

"radiance" has a transformative effect via "silent transmission." He declares that what others witness in him is really their own true nature: "The Self of the teacher and one's own Self are one and the same."

The significance of his rare state of awareness was published in an article "Beyond Reason: The Certitude of the Mystic, from Al-Hallaj to David R. Hawkins," in the *International Journal of Humanities and Social Science* (September 2011). The article gives an account of his spiritual experiences, their parallel to historical sages and saints, and their modern-day significance.[1]

Dr. Hawkins may very well be the first human being to have been trained as a modern clinical scientist/physician who has undergone the transformation classically termed "Enlightenment" or *"unio mystica"* — and then been able to contextualize the condition in lectures and books. While many of us have transient moments of "flow," intense joy, or self-transcendence, it is rare for such a state to be permanent. Historically, most such beings remain in "God-shock," unable to speak about it. As William James tells us in his classic *Varieties of Religious Experience*, the mystic experience is "ineffable."

Dr. Hawkins stands out because, following the 1965 transformation of consciousness, he dedicated himself for the next thirty years to find the means by which to communicate the ineffable spiritual truths in a way that would be comprehensible to a modern, scientific world. This book, *Power vs. Force*, is the vehicle of that communication.

The state of Enlightenment is totally complete in its bliss, such that one would never leave it except to share the gift that was given out of a total surrender of love to God and to one's fellow human beings. That

Dr. Hawkins would re-enter the world of logic and language in order to share a "map" with us so that we might also complete our destiny speaks volumes of his selfless love for humanity.

As he explained one time, "To discover something that relieves suffering — it's one's responsibility to share it with others so that they are benefited." Similar to Alexander Fleming who discovered penicillin and dedicated himself to sharing the discovery with the world, Dr. Hawkins has been dedicated to sharing the discovery of Reality in the most accessible way.

———

The information and overall context of this book hold the power to diagnose and resolve all inner blocks and ailments. It functions like an enzyme of spiritual facilitation to ameliorate suffering. Upon contact, it potentiates the inborn mechanisms of self-healing, self-awareness, and inner evolution within the human psyche.

So that the reader may see the far-reaching verification of this effect, here are representative statements given at his final public appearance in the fall of 2011:

Dr. Rev. Michael Beckwith, Founder of the Agape International Spiritual Center: "While you may think you are disappearing from the public eye, the energy frequency of your love, compassion, and wisdom remains in every heart you have touched throughout these many years. And certainly that includes my own and that of my spiritual community. You are a cosmic blessing on the planet, a beneficial presence whose imprint is deep and eternal."

Swami Chidatmananda, Hindu teacher in India: "On behalf of all the followers in India, I offer humble prostrations and respect to Dr. David Hawkins for making a great difference in all of our lives. His books make our understanding of Indian scriptures clearer, and this is true for the beginner and equally so for the advanced scholar of Sanskrit."

Dr. Marj Britt, senior minister within the Unity Church and Vice-President of its International Seminary: "I cannot thank you enough for what you have given in the world. How you have made the teachings of Jesus Christ and other masters literally come alive through your very being and your very consciousness."

Dr. Don MacDonagh, D.O., Osteopath: "I work in the medical field and have had the opportunity to see how much these ideas can help patients who are working on different issues. Once they get into this work, I know they will learn in a hundred different ways that all healing is possible for one reason only: the Love of God. On their behalf, thank you so much for your life's work and for all you've given us."

Jakob and Fabiola Merchant, speaking about the influence of his work on parenting: "We have studied your work for years, and it is the basis of our life together. It has meant that our children always remind us to forgive everybody whenever they get into trouble! More than anything, you have taught us to practice unconditional lovingness and to see the Divinity in everything, not just on an isolated mountaintop but in our everyday life."

Anonymous male, U.S.: "I spent ten years of my life in addiction, over five years shooting heroin, in and out of jails, living on the street. By the mercy of the Lord, I was exposed to your teachings in rehab a few years ago. I now live a sober life full of joy. You brought me to Christ, you brought me to Krishna, you brought me to the rooms of recovery and the 12 steps. I wake up in the morning grateful to be alive. I thought I was condemned to live the life I was living for the rest of my life, and I wake up a free man due to your grace. You saved my life."

Anonymous female, Canada: "I used to suffer from clinical depression all my life. I read *Power vs. Force*. There was a miracle. I don't suffer from panic attacks any more. I enjoy life. I am set free. I know that depression is a disease that we can't see. It's inside of us, a hole that eats us up. And I want to thank you for my freedom, for my health, and for showing me the way out of darkness."

Anonymous female, S. Korea: "The God I grew up with was a god who favored a few and was prone to rage and revenge. I could not accept such a god. Thus I was an atheist before I encountered the book *Power vs. Force*. Having no religion and spiritual knowledge of any kind, I could not answer such questions as 'Why was I born? Whence did we come and where do we go when we die?' When I was 29 years old, I discovered Dr. Hawkins' books. After that, the world wasn't the same any more. From a lifeless, black and white world sprang an exuberant and colorful world. A new life began for me."

———

The life, work, and presence of Dr. Hawkins infuse the human spirit with a new clarity and provide a trustworthy compass for the progress of our individual and collective lives.

We live in a world marked by physical, mental, and emotional suffering. What can we learn about our untapped inner resources? What exactly is the effect of a person or a group that radiates love, acceptance, and compassion? Is it really possible that our own consciousness holds the power to uplift not only ourselves but also the world? This book says, "Yes."

By showing us the way to liberation, Dr. Hawkins gives us the chance of reaching it. By contextualizing high spiritual truth into a framework that speaks to our linear, logical minds, he dissolves one of the greatest barriers to the expansion of consciousness: intellectual doubt.

As any parent knows, it takes great love to explain adult realities to the child in a way that a child can understand. This has always been the difficulty of the sage: how to communicate the nonlinear realities that lie beyond the reach of the mind in a way that the mind can understand. Dr. Hawkins demystifies the spiritual life by speaking in the idiom of our time: science. Yet with every word and reverent gesture, he preserves the utter mystery of the Absolute.

He speaks as an ordinary person to his fellows about ordinary human life. He does not don special robes, perform special ceremonies, or teach special chants or practices. As he says:

> *The truth of one's Self can be discovered in everyday life. To live with care and kindness is all that is necessary. The rest reveals itself in due time. The common-place and God are not distinct.*

He affirms the beauty of everyday life and the sacredness of each interaction: "Our love for each other is not different than our love for God."

The radical Reality is: to understand the essence of anything is to know God.

Fran Grace, Ph.D., editor

Professor of Religious Studies and
Steward of Meditation Room
University of Redlands, California
Founding Director, Institute for Contemplative Life
Sedona, Arizona

December 2011

NEW PREFACE

Since the original publication of this book, there have been a hundred presentations worldwide, to further clarify and delineate the subject matter.

The book transmits hope. It defines certainty in contrast to guesswork. It introduces the possibility of self-verification.

In daily life, it can take years for an error to show up and be rectified, often at great financial cost as well as the cost of time and energy. A million dollars and many years are spent on a project to find out whether it is even feasible, whereas one could find out the answer in a matter of seconds. So the method described in this book is highly pragmatic.

The world is interested in what sounds good which, in practice, can be disastrous. It is important to differentiate essence from appearance. Things that appear attractive end up falling apart. Things that appear mundane prove to be the supportive reality behind the effort.

Gloria in Excelsis Deo!

David R. Hawkins, M.D., Ph.D.
Founding Director
Institute for Spiritual Research
Sedona, Arizona

December 2011

MISIDENTIFIES
HIS OWN INTELLECTUAL
ARTIFACTS AS REALITY

INTRODUCTION

COMMON UNSTATED GOAL — UNDERSTANDING OR INFLUENCING HUMAN EXPERIENCE

All human endeavor has the common, unstated goal of understanding or influencing human experience. To this end, man has developed numerous descriptive and analytical disciplines: morality, philosophy, psychology, and so forth. Staggering amounts of time and money are invested in data collection and analysis in attempts to predict human trends. Implicit in this frenetic search is the expectation of finding some ultimate "answer." The "answer," we seem perennially to believe, will, once found, allow us to solve the problems of the economy, crime, national health, or politics. But so far, we have solved none.

It is not that we lack data—we are virtually drowning in data. The obstacle is that we do not have the proper tools to interpret the significance of our data. We have not yet asked the right questions because we have not had an adequate gauge of our questions' relevance or accuracy. Man's dilemma— now and always—has been that he misidentifies his own intellectual artifacts as reality.[1] But these artificial suppositions are merely the products of an arbitrary point of perception. The inadequacy of the answers we receive is a direct consequence of the limitations implicit in the viewpoints of the questioner. Slight errors in the formation of questions result in gross errors in the answers that follow.

Understanding does not proceed simply from examining data; it comes from examining data in a particular context. Data is useless until we know what it *means*. To understand its meaning, we need not only

xlix

to ask the right question; we also need the appropriate instruments with which to measure the data in a meaningful process of sorting and description.

Most of human behavior has remained indecipherable despite all attempts to understand it in depth. The systems we have created to achieve understanding may seem extensive and impressive, but each in turn has led us down a blind alley because of limitations inherent in the original design. As we explore the nature of man's problems, it becomes clear that there has never been a reliable experimental yardstick with which to measure and interpret man's motivations and experiences over the course of history.

Philosophy in all of its branches attempts to comprehend human experience by creating abstractions and hypothecating their concordance with some ultimate reality. Political systems are all based on suppositions about relative human values lacking any demonstrable factual basis. All systems of morality resolve into arbitrary attempts to reduce the enormous complexities of human behavior to simplistic categories of right and wrong. Psychoanalysis, in exposing the unconscious mind, has compounded this muddle, giving rise to a bewildering array of treatments and psychologies derived from various viewpoints. This ongoing babble of man's attempt to understand himself finally produces a semantic morass in which, in the end, anything one might say is probably true to some degree. Because of uncertainty about the exact nature of causality, even when measurable results are obtained, they are subject to being ascribed to factitious causes.

The fatal faults of all thought systems have been, primarily: (1) failure to differentiate between subjective

1

and objective; (2) disregard of the limitation of context inherent in basic design and terminology; (3) ignorance of the nature of consciousness itself; and (4) misunderstanding of the nature of causality. The consequences of these shortcomings will become obvious as we explore the major areas of human experience from a new perspective, with new tools.

Society constantly expends its efforts to correct effects instead of causes, which is one reason why the evolution of human consciousness proceeds so slowly. Mankind is really barely on the first rung of the ladder; we have not yet solved even such primitive problems as world hunger. The accomplishments of mankind, in fact, thus far are most impressive for having been achieved—almost blindly—through trial and error. While this random search for solutions has resulted in a maze of baffling complexity, true answers always have the hallmark of simplicity. The basic law of the universe is economy. The universe does not waste a single quark; all serves a purpose and fits into a balance—there are no extraneous events.

Man is stuck with his lack of knowledge about himself until he can learn to look beyond apparent causes. From the human record, we may note that answers never arise from identifying so-called "causes" in the world. Instead, it is necessary to identify the conditions that underlie ostensible causes; and these conditions exist only within man's consciousness itself. No definitive answer to any problem can be found by isolating sequences of events and projecting upon them a mental notion of "causality." There are no actual causes within the observable world. As we shall demonstrate, the observable world is a world of effects.

What is the human prognosis? Is society by virtue of its own chaotic subsystems a runaway juggernaut, inherently doomed? This prospect underlies a general social apprehension about the future. International polls indicate a high level of unhappiness everywhere on the globe, even in the most advanced countries.[2] While the majority of people resign themselves to a pessimistic view and pray for a better life in the "hereafter," the few visionaries who foresee a utopian future are unable to describe the means necessary to bring it about. Society needs *visionaries of means, not dreamers of ends.* Once we have the means, the ends will reveal themselves.

The difficulty in finding effective means reduces itself, upon examination, to our inability to discriminate the essential from the nonessential. Thus far, there has been no system affording a method by which to distinguish powerful and effective solutions from weak, ineffective ones. Our means of evaluation themselves have been inherently incapable of performing realistic appraisal.

Societal choices, more often than not, are the result of expediency, statistical fallacy, sentiment, political or media pressure, or personal prejudice and vested interest. Crucial decisions affecting the lives of everyone on the planet are made under conditions that virtually guarantee failure. Because societies lack the necessary reality base for formulation of effective problem resolutions, they fall back, over and over, on a resort to force (in its various expressions—such as war, law, taxation, rules, and regulations), which is extremely costly, instead of employing power, which is very economical.

Man's two basic types of operational faculties, reason and feeling, are both inherently unreliable, as our history of precarious individual and collective survival attests. Although we ascribe our actions to reason, man in fact operates primarily out of pattern-recognition; the logical arrangement of data serves mainly to enhance a pattern-recognition system that then becomes so-called "truth."[3] But nothing is ever "true," except under certain circumstances, and then only from a particular viewpoint, characteristically unstated.

As a result, thoughtful man deduces that all of his problems arise from the difficulty of "knowingness." Ultimately, the mind arrives at epistemology, the branch of philosophy that examines the question of how and to what degree man really knows anything. Such philosophical discussions may seem either erudite or irrelevant, but the questions they pose are at the very core of human experience. No matter where we start in an examination of human knowledge, we always end up looking at the phenomena of awareness and the nature of human consciousness. And we eventually come to the same realization: any further advance in man's condition requires a verifiable basis for knowingness, upon which we may place our trust.

The main obstacle to man's development, then, is the lack of knowledge about the nature of consciousness itself. If we look within ourselves at the instant-by-instant processes of our minds, we will soon notice that the mind acts much more rapidly than we would acknowledge. It becomes apparent that the notion that our actions are based on thoughtful decisions is a grand illusion. The decision-making process is a function of consciousness itself; with enormous rapidity, the mind makes choices based on millions of pieces of data and their correlations and projections, far beyond conscious comprehension. This is a global function dominated by the energy patterns that the new science of nonlinear dynamics terms *attractors*.[4]

Consciousness automatically chooses what it deems best from instant to instant because that is ultimately the only function of which it is really capable. The relative weight and merit given to certain data are determined by a predominant attractor pattern operating in the individual or in a collective group of minds. These patterns can be identified, described, and calibrated; out of that information arises a totally new understanding of human behavior, history, and the potential destiny of mankind.

The present volume, the result of twenty years of intensive research involving millions of calibrations, can make such understanding available to anyone. That this revelation proceeds from a fortuitous connection between the physiology of consciousness, the function of the human nervous system, and the physics of the universe is not surprising when we remind ourselves that we are, after all, part of a universe in which everything is connected to everything else; all its secrets are thus, theoretically at least, available to us if we know where and how to look.

Can man lift himself up by his bootstraps? Why not? All he has to do is increase his buoyancy and he will effortlessly rise to a higher state. Force cannot accomplish that feat; power not only can, but constantly does.

Man thinks he lives by virtue of the forces he can control, but in fact, he is governed by power from unrevealed sources, power over which he has no control. Because power is effortless, it goes unseen and unsuspected. Force is experienced through the senses; power can be recognized only through inner awareness. Man is immobilized in his present condition by his alignment with enormously powerful attractor energy patterns, which he himself unconsciously sets in motion. Moment by moment, he is suspended in this state of evolution, restrained by the energies of force, impelled by the energies of power.

The individual is thus like a cork in the sea of consciousness—he does not know where he is, where he came from, or where he is going, and he does not know why. Man wanders about in this endless conundrum, asking the same questions century after century, and so he will continue, failing a quantum leap in consciousness. One mark of such a sudden expansion of context and understanding is an inner experience of relief, joy, and awe. All who have had such an experience feel afterwards that the universe has granted them a precious gift. Facts are accumulated by effort, but truth reveals itself effortlessly.[5]

Hopefully, through this book, the reader can comprehend and then prepare the conditions for such a personal revelation; to do so is the ultimate adventure.

PART ONE: TOOLS

CHAPTER 1

Critical Advances in Knowledge

The evolution of this work, which began in 1965, was fostered by developments in numerous scientific fields—of which three were of special importance. Clinical research on the physiology of the nervous system and the holistic functioning of the human organism resulted in the development in the 1970s of the new science of *kinesiology*.[1] Meanwhile, in the technological arena, computers were being designed that were capable of millions of calculations in milliseconds, making possible the new tools of artificial intelligence.[2] This abrupt access to formerly inconceivable masses of data begat a revolutionary perspective on natural phenomena: *chaos theory*. Simultaneously, in the theoretical sciences, quantum mechanics led to advanced theoretical physics; through associated mathematics, a whole new study of *nonlinear dynamics* emerged—this was one of the most far-reaching developments of modern science, the long-term impact of which has yet to be realized.[3]

Kinesiology exposed, for the first time, the intimate connection between mind and body, revealing that the mind "thinks" with the body itself. Thence, it provided an avenue for the exploration of the ways consciousness reveals itself in the subtle mechanisms behind disease processes.[4]

Advanced computers, permitting the depiction through graphics of vast amounts of data, disclosed unsuspected systems within what had been ignored by Newtonian physics as indecipherable or meaningless, chaotic data.[5] Theoreticians in diverse fields were suddenly able to intimate coherent ways of understanding data that had been considered incoherent or *nonlinear*—diffuse, or chaotic, and therefore inaccessible through conventional probabilistic logical theory and mathematics.

Analysis of this seemingly "incoherent" data identified hidden energy patterns, or *attractors* (which had been postulated by the advanced mathematics of nonlinear equations). These existed behind apparently random natural phenomena.[6] Computer graphics clearly demonstrated the designs of these attractor fields. The implicit potential for analyzing supposedly unpredictable systems in such disparate areas as fluid mechanics, human biology, and stellar astronomy appeared to be limitless. (The public, however, has remained generally unaware of the field of nonlinear dynamics, except for the appearance in the marketplace of some intriguing new computer graphics patterns generated by "fractal" geometry.)

During the era preceding these revelations, linear science had grown progressively divorced from concern with the basis of life itself—all life processes are, in fact, nonlinear. This isolation was also characteristic of medicine, which, when presented with the amazing discoveries of kinesiology, merely ignored the information because it had no context, no paradigm of reality, with which to comprehend it. Medicine had forgotten that it was an art, and that science was merely a tool of that art.

Within medicine, psychiatry had always been held at a distance by traditionalists because it dealt with the immeasurables of human life and therefore appeared less "scientific"- that is, from the Newtonian view-point Academic psychiatry, in fact, has made major scientific breakthroughs in psychopharmacology since at least the 1950s. However, it remains the most nonlinear area of medicine, examining such subjects as intuition, decision-making, and the whole phenomenon of life as process Although in the academic psychiatric literature there is little mention of such things as love, meaning, value, or will, the psychiatric discipline at least essays a somewhat larger view of man than other traditional medical fields.

———•———

Regardless of what branch of inquiry one starts from—philosophy, political theory, theology, etc.—all avenues of investigation eventually converge at a common meeting point: the quest for an organized understanding of the nature of pure consciousness. But all of the major enterprises in human knowledge discussed above—even kinesiology and nonlinear dynamics—halted at this last great barrier to human knowledge, the investigation of the nature of consciousness itself. Some advanced thinkers, it is true, went beyond the parameters of their respective fields and began to ask questions about the relationship between the universe, science, and consciousness in its experience as mind.[7] We will refer to their theories and their impact on the advance of human understanding as we proceed.

The thesis of the present work derives from amalgamating these several scientific disciplines into a methodology both elegantly simple and rewarding. We have thereby found that consciousness can indeed be investigated. Although no road maps for such a study have thus far been available, research into the subject has produced its own design, and with it, the context needed to comprehend its findings.

Inasmuch as everything in the universe is connected with everything else,[8] it is not surprising that one of the primary objectives of this study—a map of the energy fields of consciousness—would correlate with, and be corroborated by, all other avenues of investigation, uniting the diversity of human experience and its expressions in an all-encompassing paradigm.[9] Such an insight can bypass the artificial dichotomy between subject and object, transcending the limited viewpoint that creates the illusion of duality. The subjective and objective are, in fact, one and the same,[10] as can be demonstrated without resorting to nonlinear equations or computer graphics.

By identifying subjective and objective as the same, we are able to transcend the constraints of the concept of time, which by its very definition is a major hindrance to comprehension of the nature of life, especially in its expression as human experience. If, in actuality, the so-called subjective and objective are really one and the same, then we can find the answers to all questions by merely looking within man himself. By simply recording observations, we can see a grand picture emerge, one that predicates no limitations to the extent of further investigation.

All of us have available at all times a computer far more advanced than the most elaborate artificial intelligence machine—the human mind itself. The basic function of any measuring device is simply to give a

ARTIFICIAL DICOTOMY BETWEEN SUBJECTIVE + OBJECTIVE

signal indicating the detection by the instrument of a slight change. In the experiments to be described in this book, the reactions of the human body itself provide such a signal of change in conditions. As will be seen, the body can discern, to the finest degree, the difference between that which is supportive of life and that which is not.

We should not be surprised at this. Living things all react to what is life-supportive and what is not; this is the fundamental mechanism of survival. Inherent in all life forms is the capacity to detect change and react correctively—thus, trees become smaller at higher elevations as the oxygen in the atmosphere becomes scarcer. Human protoplasm is far more sensitive than that of a tree.

The methodology, proceeding from the study of nonlinear dynamics, which we employed in this work of developing a map of the fields of human consciousness, is known as *attractor research*. It is concerned with the identification of power ranges of energy fields utilizing *critical point analysis*.[11] (Critical point analysis is a technique derived from the fact that in any highly complex system there is a specific, critical point at which the smallest input will result in the greatest change. For instance, the great gears of a windmill can be halted by lightly touching the right escape mechanism, and it is possible to paralyze a giant locomotive if you know exactly where to put your finger.)

Nonlinear dynamics enables these significant patterns to be identified in complex presentations, even when they are obscured by incoherence or sheer mass of indecipherable data. It discovers the relevance in what the world discards as irrelevant, using an entirely different approach and totally different methods of problem resolution from the ones the world is used to.[12]

The world conventionally assumes that the processing of problems requires starting from the known (the question or conditions) and moving on to the unknown (the so-called answer) in a time sequence following definite steps and logical progression. Nonlinear dynamics moves in the opposite direction: from the unknown (the nondeterministic data of the question) to the known (the answer)! It operates within a different paradigm of causality. The problem is seen as one of definition and access rather than of logical sequence (as in solving a problem by differential equations).[13]

DEFINITION & ACCESS RATHER THAN LOGICAL SEQUENCE

But before we attempt to define the questions of this study further, let us examine some of the material we have introduced in greater detail.

Attractors

Attractor is the name given to an identifiable pattern that emerges from a seemingly unmeaningful mass of data. There is a hidden coherence in all that appears incoherent. This inner coherence was first demonstrated in nature by Edward Lorenz in studying computer graphics derived from weather patterns over long courses of time. The attractor pattern he identified is now quite famous as "Lorenz's Butterfly."

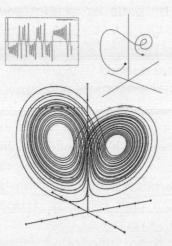

Different types of attractors are denoted by different names, for instance, *strange attractors*. But most important to our research is the discovery that some patterns are very powerful and others are much weaker. There is a critical point that differentiates the two distinct classes. This phenomenon is parallel and corollary to the high and low energy bonds in the mathematics of the chemical bond.

Fields of Dominance
A field of dominance is exhibited by high-energy patterns in their influence over weaker ones. This may be likened to the coexistence of a small magnetic field within the much larger, more powerful field of a giant electromagnet. The phenomenological universe is the expression of the interaction of endless attractor patterns of varying strengths. The unending complexities of life are the reflections of the endless reverberations of the augmentations and diminutions of these fields,

compounded by their harmonics and other interactions.

Critical Point Analysis

The traditional Newtonian concept of causality (see below) had excluded all such "nondeterministic" data because such information did not fit into its paradigm. With the discoveries of Einstein, Heisenberg, Bell, Bohr, and others, our model of the universe expanded rapidly. Advanced theoretical physics demonstrated that everything in the universe is subtly dependent upon and interactive with everything else.[14]

The classic Newtonian four-dimensional universe is often described as a giant clockworks, with the three dimensions of space manifesting linear processes in time. If we look at even simpler clockworks, we will notice that some gears move slowly and ponderously, while others move very rapidly, and tiny balances twirl about as escape mechanisms seesaw back and forth. To place pressure on one of the large moving gears would have little effect on the mechanism; however, somewhere there is a delicate balance mechanism at which point the slightest touch stops the entire device. This is identified as the "critical point," where the least force exerts the greatest effect.

Causality

Within the observable world, causality has conventionally been presumed to work in the following manner:

$$A \rightarrow B \rightarrow C$$

This is called a deterministic linear sequence—like billiard balls sequentially striking each other. The implicit presumption is that A causes B causes C.

But our own research indicates that causality operates in a completely different manner, in which the attractor pattern complex "ABC" splits through its "operants" and is expressed as the seeming sequence "A, then B, then C" of perception.

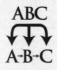

From this diagram we see that the source (ABC), which is unobservable, results in the visible sequence A→B→C, which is an observable phenomenon within the measurable three-dimensional world. The typical problems the world attempts to deal with exist on the observable level of A→B→C. But our work is to find the inherent attractor pattern, the ABC out of which the A→B→C seems to arise.

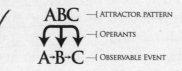

In this simple diagram, the operants transcend both the observable and the non-observable; we might picture them as a rainbow bridging the deterministic and the nondeterministic realms. (The existence of so-called operants can be inferred by asking the question, "What encompasses both the possible and the impossible, the known and the unknown?" In other words, what is the matrix of all possibilities?)

This description of how the universe works is in accord with the theories of ~~physicist~~ David Bohm, who has described a holographic universe with an invisible implicate ("enfolded") and a manifest explicate ("unfolded") order.[15] But it is most important to note that this scientific insight corresponds with the view of reality experienced through history by enlightened sages who have evolved beyond consciousness to the state of pure awareness.[16] Bohm postulates a source that is beyond both the explicate and implicate realms, very much like the state of pure awareness described by the sages.[17]

The advent of artificial intelligence supercomputers has allowed the application of the theories of nonlinear dynamics to be applied to the study of brain function through the technique of *neurophysiologic modeling*.[18] The function of memory is especially being studied by means of neural models, among which attractor networks have been identified. Conclusions of current research are that the brain's neural networks ~~act as a system of attractor patterns,~~ so that the system ~~does not behave in a random fashion~~ overall—although each individual neuron may behave in seemingly random fashion.[19]

Neuron models of consciousness disclose a class of neural networks called "constraint satisfaction systems."[20] In these systems, a network of interconnected neuron units operates within a series of limits and ~~thus sets up attractor patterns,~~ some of which are now being identified with psycho-pathology.[21] This kind of

CONSTRAINT SATISFACTION SYSTEMS.

PHASE SPACE

modeling correlates behavior with physiology and parallels the results of our kinesiologic muscle testing, demonstrating the connection between mind and body.

In terms derived from *chaos theory*, the clinical study described in the following pages has identified a *phase space*, encompassing the full range of the evolution of human consciousness. Within this range, numerous attractor patterns of increasing power have been denoted. These patterns represent energy fields that are qualities of consciousness itself rather than of any particular individual, as is shown by their occurrence across large populations over long periods of time, independent of testers or subjects.

The evolution of consciousness and the development of human society can be depicted in the mathematical terms of nonlinear dynamics. Our study concerned itself with a limited set of parameters of consciousness that we calibrated from 1 to 1,000. The numbers represent the logarithm (to the base 10) of the power of the respective fields. The entire field or phase space of consciousness itself is unlimited, going on up to infinity. The range of 1 to 600, representing the domain of the vast majority of human experience, is the primary scope of this study; the levels from 600 to 1,000, the realm of non-ordinary evolution—that of enlightenment, sages, and the highest spiritual states—will later be described.

Within the total field studied, sequential patterns emerged identifying the progressive powers of attractor fields in which there were local variations, but global consistency. So-called "strange attractors" can be of either high or low energy, and the critical point in our data appeared to be the calibration level of 200, below which the power of attractors could be described as weak or negative, above which as strong or positive. By the time we reached the calibration of 600, they were enormously powerful.

An important element of chaos theory, which is helpful in understanding this evolution of consciousness, is the *law of sensitive dependence on initial conditions*.[22] This refers to the fact that a slight variation over a course of time can have the effect of producing a profound change,[23] much as a ship whose bearing is one degree off compass will eventually find itself hundreds of miles off course. This phenomenon, which we will refer to in more detail later, is an essential mechanism of all evolution and also underlies the potential of the creative process.

———

In overview, we can see that from time immemorial, man has tried to make sense of the enormous complexity and frequent unpredictability of human behavior. A multitude of systems has been constructed to try to make that which is incomprehensible comprehensible. To "make sense" has ordinarily meant to be definable in terms that are linear: logical and rational. But the process, and therefore the experience, of life itself, is organic—that is to say, nonlinear by definition. This is the source of man's inescapable intellectual frustration.

In this study, however, test responses were independent of our subjects' belief systems or intellectual content. What emerged were patterns of energy fields that were aspects of consciousness itself, irrespective of individual identities. In common left-brain/right-brain parlance, we could say that the test subjects reacted globally to an attractor field, irrespective of the individual variation of their left-brain logic, reason, or sequential thought systems. The results of the study indicate that profoundly powerful patterns organize human behavior.

We can intuit, then, an infinite domain of infinite potential—consciousness itself—within which there is an enormously powerful attractor Field organizing all of human behavior into what is innate to "humanness." Within the giant attractor Field are lesser Fields of progressively less energy and power. These Fields, in turn, dominate behavior, so that definable patterns are consistent across cultures and time, throughout human history. The interactions of these variations within attractor Fields make up the history of civilization and mankind. (A side study not herein reported indicated that the animal and vegetable kingdoms are also controlled by attractor Fields of hierarchic power.)

Our study correlates well with Rupert Sheldrake's "morphogenetic fields" hypothesis, as well as with Karl Pribram's holographic model of brain-mind function.[24] (Note that in a holographic universe, the achievements of every individual contribute to the advancement and well-being of the whole.) Our study also correlates with the conclusions reached by Nobelist Sir John Eccles that the brain acts as a receiving set for energy patterns residing within the mind itself, which exist as consciousness expressed in the form of thought.[25] It is the vanity of the ego that claims thoughts as "mine." Genius, on the other hand, commonly attributes the source of creative leaps of awareness to that basis of all consciousness, which has traditionally been called Divinity.

CHAPTER 2

History and Methodology

The basis of this work is research done over a twenty-year period, involving millions of calibrations on thousands of test subjects of all ages and personality types, and from all walks of life. By design, the study is clinical in method and thus has widespread, pragmatic implications. Because this testing method is valid in application to all forms of human expression, calibrations have successfully been taken for literature, architecture, art, science, world events, and the complexities of human relationships. The test space for the determination of the data is the totality of the human experience throughout all time.

Mentally, test subjects ranged from what the world calls "normal" to severely ill psychiatric patients. Subjects were tested in Canada, the United States, Mexico, and throughout South America, and Northern Europe. They were of all nationalities, ethnic backgrounds, and religions, ranging in age from children to elders in their nineties, and covered a wide spectrum of physical and emotional health. Subjects were tested individually and in groups by many different testers and groups of testers. In general, the results were identical and reproducible, fulfilling the fundamental requirement of the scientific method: perfect experimental replicability.[1]

Subjects were selected at random and tested in a wide array of physical and behavioral settings: on top of mountains and at the seashore, at holiday parties and during the course of everyday work, in moments of joy

73

and moments of sorrow. None of these circumstances affected the test results, which were found to be universally consistent irrespective of extraneous factors, with the singular exception of the methodology of the testing procedure itself. Because of the significance of this factor, the testing method will be described in detail below.

Historical Background

In 1971, three physiotherapists published a definitive study on muscle-testing.[2] Dr. George Goodheart, of Detroit, Michigan, had studied muscle-testing techniques extensively in his clinical practice and made the breakthrough discovery that the strength or weakness of every muscle was connected to the health or pathology of a specific corresponding body organ.[3] He further determined that each individual muscle was associated with an acupuncture meridian and correlated his work with that of the physician Felix Mann on the medical significance of the acupuncture meridians.[4]

By 1976, Dr. Goodheart's book on applied kinesiology had reached its 12th edition; he began to teach the technique to his colleagues and also published monthly research tapes. His work was rapidly picked up by others, which led to the formation of the International College of Applied Kinesiology, many members of which also belonged to the Academy of Preventive Medicine. A thorough exposition of the development of the field was detailed by David Walther in his extensive volume on applied kinesiology, also published in 1976.[5]

The most striking finding of kinesiology initially

was a clear demonstration that muscles instantly become weak when the body is exposed to harmful stimuli. For instance, if a patient with hypoglycemia put sugar on his tongue, upon muscle testing, the deltoid muscle (the one usually used as an indicator muscle) instantly went weak. Accordingly, it was discovered that substances that were therapeutic to the body made the muscles instantly become strong.

Because the weakness of any particular muscle indicated the presence of a pathologic process in its corresponding organ (corroborated by diagnosis through acupuncture and physical or laboratory examination), it was a highly useful clinical tool to detect disease. Thousands of practitioners began to use the method, and data rapidly accumulated showing kinesiology to be an important and reliable diagnostic technique that could accurately monitor a patient's response to treatment as well as diagnosis.

The technique found widespread acceptance among professionals from many disciplines, and although it never caught on in mainstream medicine, it was used extensively by holistically oriented physicians. One of these was Dr. John Diamond, a psychiatrist who began to use kinesiology in diagnosing and treating psychiatric patients. He labeled this extended use of kinesiology as "behavioral kinesiology."[6]

While other investigators were researching the usefulness of the method in detecting allergies, nutritional disorders, and responses to medications, Dr. Diamond used the technique to research the beneficial or adverse effects of a great variety of sensory and psychological stimuli, such as art forms, music, facial expression, voice modulation, and emotional stress. He was an excellent teacher, and his seminars attracted thousands of professionals who returned to their own practices with renewed interest and curiosity as they explored applications of the technique.

In addition to its inclusive applicability, the test was quick, simple, easy to perform, and highly decisive; all researchers confirmed the replicability of test results. For example, an artificial sweetener made every subject test weak, whether placed on the tongue, held in its package adjacent to the solar plexus, or hidden in a plain envelope (the contents of which neither the tester nor the subject knew).

That the body responded even when the mind was naïve was most impressive. Most practitioners did their own verification research, placing various substances in plain, numbered envelopes and having a naïve second person test a third. The overwhelming conclusion was that the body would indeed respond accurately, even when the conscious mind was unaware.

The reliability of the testing experience never ceased to amaze the public and patients—and, for that matter, the practitioners themselves. When this author was on the lecture circuit, in audiences of 1,000 people, 500 envelopes containing artificial sweetener would be passed out to the audience, along with 500 identical envelopes containing organic vitamin C. The audience would then be divided up and would alternate testing each other. When the envelopes were opened, the audience reaction was always one of amazement and delight when they saw that everybody had gone weak in response to the artificial sweetener and strong in response to the organic vitamin C. The nutritional habits of thousands of families across the country were changed by this simple demonstration.

In the early 1970s, the medical profession in general, and psychiatry in particular, was highly resistant—if not forthrightly hostile—to the idea that nutrition had much to do with health at all, let alone emotional health or brain function. Publication of the book *Orthomolecular Psychiatry*, by this author and Nobelist Linus Pauling, received a favorable reception from a wide variety of audiences, but not from the medical establishment.[7] (Interestingly enough, more than twenty years later, the concepts presented in the book are now fundamental to the current treatment of mental illness.)

The thrust of this book was that serious mental illnesses such as psychosis, as well as lesser ones, such as emotional disorder, had a genetic basis involving an abnormal biochemical pathway in the brain, a molecular basis that could be corrected on the molecular level. Manic-depressive illness, schizophrenia, alcoholism, and depression, therefore, could be affected by nutrition as well as medication. In 1973, when *Orthomolecular Psychiatry* was published, the psychiatric establishment was still psychoanalytically oriented; the work was primarily accepted by holistic practitioners. The suggested treatment methods and results were frequently verified with kinesiology.

However, it was Dr. Diamond's demonstration that the body instantly went weak in response to unhealthy emotional attitudes or mental stresses that had the greatest ongoing clinical influence. His refinement of

the muscle-testing technique, the one used by most
practitioners, was used in this study over a period of
twenty years. It was universally observed by practitioners
and researchers, as well as by this author, that test
responses were completely independent of the test
subjects' belief systems, intellectual opinions, reason, or
logic. It was also observed that a test response where
the subject went weak was accompanied by desynchronization of the cerebral hemispheres.[8]

The Testing Technique
Two persons are required. One acts as test subject by
holding out one arm laterally, parallel to the ground.
The second person then presses down with two fingers on the wrist of the extended arm and says, "Resist."
The subject then resists the downward pressure with
all his strength. That is all there is to it.

A statement may be made by either party. While the
subject holds it in mind, his arm's strength is tested by
the tester's downward pressure. If the statement is negative, false, or reflects a calibration below 200 (see
"Map of Consciousness," Chapter 3), the test subject
will "go weak." If the answer is yes or calibrates over
200, he will "go strong."

To demonstrate the procedure, one might have the
subject hold an image of Abraham Lincoln in mind
while being tested, and then, for contrast, an image of
Adolf Hitler. The same effect can be demonstrated by
holding in mind someone who is loved in contrast to
someone who is feared, hated, or about whom there is
some strong regret.

Once a numeric scale is elicited (see below) calibrations can be arrived at by stating, "This item" (such as this book, organization, this person's motive, and so on) calibrates "over 100," then "over 200," then "over 300," until a negative response is obtained. The calibration can then be refined: "It is over 220. 225. 230.," and so on. Tester and testee can trade places, and the same results will be obtained. Once one is familiar with the technique, it can be used to evaluate companies, movies, individuals, or events in history; it can also be used to diagnose current life problems.

The test procedure, the reader will note, is to use the muscle test to verify the truth or falsity of a declarative statement. Unreliable responses will be obtained if the question has not been put into this form. Nor can a reliable result be obtained from inquiry into the future; only statements regarding existent conditions or events in the past or present will produce consistent answers.

It is necessary to be impersonal during the procedure to avoid transmitting positive or negative feelings. Accuracy is increased by having the test subject close his eyes, and there should be no music or distractions in the background.

Because the test is so deceptively simple, it is well that inquirers first verify its accuracy to their own satisfaction. Responses can be checked by cross-questioning, and everyone who becomes acquainted with the technique thinks of tricks to satisfy themselves that it is reliable.[9] It will soon be found that the same response is observed in all subjects, that it is not necessary for the subject to have any knowledge of the matter in question, and that the response will always be independent of the test subject's personal opinions about the question.

Before presenting an inquiry, we have found that it is useful to first test the statement, "I have permission to ask this question." This is analogous to an entry requisite on a computer terminal, and will occasionally return a "no" answer. This indicates that one should leave that question alone or inquire carefully into the reason for the "no." Perhaps the questioner might have experienced psychological distress from the answer or its implications at that time, or for other unknown reasons.[10]

In this study, test subjects were asked to focus on a specified thought, feeling, attitude, memory, relationship, or life circumstance. The test was frequently done in large groups of people; for demonstration purposes, we first established a baseline by asking the subjects, eyes closed, to hold in mind the memory of a time when they were angry, upset, jealous, depressed, guilty, or fearful; at that point, everyone universally went weak. We would then ask them to hold in mind a loving person or life situation, and everyone would go strong; typically a murmur of surprise would ripple through the audience at the implications of what they had just discovered.

The next phenomenon demonstrated was that the mere image of a substance held in the mind produced the same response as if the substance itself were in physical contact with the body. As an example, we would hold up an apple grown with pesticides and ask the audience to look directly at it while being tested; all would go weak. We would then hold up an organically grown apple, free of contaminants, and as the audience focused on it, they would instantly go strong. Inasmuch as no one in the audience knew which apple was which, nor, for that matter, had any anticipation of the test at all, the reliability of the method was demonstrated to everyone's satisfaction.[11]

For reliable results, it should be remembered that people process experience differently; some people primarily adopt a feeling mode, others are more auditory, and still others are more visual. Therefore, test questions should avoid such phrasing as "How do you feel?" about a person, situation, or experience; or "How does it look?" or "How does it sound?" Customarily, if one says, "Hold the situation (or person, place, thing, or feeling) in mind," the subjects will instinctively select their own appropriate mode.[12]

Occasionally, in an effort, perhaps even unconscious, to disguise their response, subjects will select a mode that is not their customary mode of processing and give a false response. When the tester elicits a paradoxical response, the question should be rephrased. For example, a patient who feels guilty about his anger toward his mother may hold in mind a photograph of her and test strong. However, if the tester were to rephrase the question by asking this subject to hold in mind his present attitude toward his mother, the subject would instantly go weak.

Other precautions to maintain the accuracy of the test include removing eyeglasses, especially if they have metal frames, and hats (synthetic materials on top of the head make everyone go weak). The testing arm should also be free of jewelry, especially quartz wristwatches. When an anomalous response does occur, further investigation will eventually reveal the cause— the tester, for instance, might be wearing a perfume to which the patient has an adverse reaction, producing false negative responses. If a tester experiences repeated failures while attempting to elicit an accurate response, the effect of his voice on other subjects should be evaluated; some testers, at least at certain times, may express sufficient negative energy in their voices to affect test results.[13]

Another factor to be considered in the face of a paradoxical response is the time frame of the memory or image involved. If a test subject is holding in mind a given person and their relationship, the response will depend on the period the memory or image represents. If he is remembering his relationship with his brother from childhood, he may have a different response than if he is holding in mind an image of the relationship as it is today. Questioning always has to be narrowed down specifically.[14]

One other cause for paradoxical test results is a physical condition of the test subject resulting from stress, or depression of the thymus gland function, which occurs from encountering a very negative energy field. The thymus gland is the central controller of the body's acupuncture energy system, and when its energy is low, test results are unpredictable. This can be easily remedied in a few seconds by a simple technique discovered by Dr. John Diamond, which he called the "thymic thump." The thymus gland is located directly behind the top of the breastbone. With clenched fist, pound over this area rhythmically several times while smiling and thinking of someone you love. At each thump, say, "Ha-ha-ha." Retesting will now show the resumption of thymic dominance, and normal test results will occur.[15]

Use of the Testing Procedure in This Study

The testing technique just described is that recommended by Dr. Diamond in *Behavioral Kinesiology*. The only variation introduced in our study was the correlation of responses with a logarithmic scale to calibrate the relative power of the energy of different attitudes, thoughts, feelings, situations, and relationships. Because the test is rapid, actually taking less than ten seconds, it is possible to process an enormous amount of information about a variety of matters in a very short time.

The numerical scale elicited spontaneously from test subjects ranges from the value of mere physical existence at 1, up to 600 in the ordinary worldly realm, which is the apex of ordinary consciousness, and then from 600 on up to 1,000, which includes advanced states of enlightenment. Responses in the form of simple yes-or-no answers determine the calibration of the subject. For example, "If just being alive is one, then the power of love is over 200." (Subject goes strong, indicating a yes.) "Love is over 300." (Subject still goes strong.) "Love is over 400." (Subject stays strong.) "Love is 500 or over." (Subject still strong.) In this case, love calibrated at 500, and this figure proved reproducible regardless of how many subjects were tested. With repeated testing—using either individuals or groups— a consistent scale emerged, which correlates well with human experience, history, and common opinion, as well as the findings of psychology, sociology, psycho-analysis, philosophy, medicine, and the famous Great Chain of Being. It also correlates quite precisely with Perennial Philosophy's "strata of consciousness."[16]

The tester must be cautious, however, realizing that the answers to some questions may be quite disturbing to the subject. The technique must not be used irresponsibly and the tester must always respect the subject's willingness to participate; it should never be used as a confrontational technique. In clinical situations, a personal question is never posed to the test subject unless it is pertinent to a therapeutic purpose. It is possible, though, to pose a question that precludes personal involvement on the part of the test subject, who then functions merely as an indicator for the purposes of calibration research.

The test response is independent of the subject's actual physical strength. It is frequently dumbfounding to well-muscled athletes when they go just as weak as anyone else in response to a noxious stimulus. The tester may well be a frail woman who weighs less than 100 pounds, and the subject may be a professional football player who weighs more than 200, but the test results will be the same, as she puts down his powerful arm with a mere two fingers.

Discrepancies
Differing calibrations may be obtained over time or by different investigators for a variety of reasons:

1. Situations, people, politics, policies, and attitudes change over time.

2. People tend to use different sensory modalities when they hold something in mind, i.e., visual, sensory, auditory, or feeling. "Your mother" could therefore be how she looked, felt, sounded, etc., or Henry Ford could be calibrated as a father, as an industrialist, for his impact on America, his anti-Semitism, etc.

3. Unless a specific scale is used as reference, the numbers obtained will be arbitrary. All calibrations in this book were made in reference to the Map of Consciousness (Chapter 3). For instance: "On a scale of 1 to 600 where 600 represents enlightenment, this _____ calibrates at _____." If a specific scale is not specified, testers may get astounding numbers over 1,000 and progressively higher numbers with subsequent tests. On this scale, no person who existed on this planet ever calibrated over 1,000, which is the calibration of all the Great Avatars.

One can specify context and stick to a prevailing modality. The same team using the same technique will get results that are internally consistent. Expertise develops with practice.

The best attitude is one of clinical detachment, posing a statement with the prefix statement, "In the name of the highest good, _____ calibrates as true. Over 100. Over 200., etc." The contextualization "in the highest good" increases accuracy because it transcends self-serving personal interest and motives.

There are some people, however, who are incapable

of a scientific, detached attitude and unable to be objective, and for whom the kinesiologic method will therefore not be accurate. Dedication and intention to the truth have to be given priority over personal opinions and trying to prove them as being "right."

Limitations

The test is accurate only if the test subjects themselves calibrate over 200 and the intention of the use of the test is integrous, calibrating over 200. The requirement is one of detached objectivity and alignment with truth rather than subjective opinion. Thus, to try to prove a point negates accuracy. Approximately 10% of the population is not able to use the kinesiologic testing technique for as yet unknown reasons. Sometimes married couples, also for reasons as yet undiscovered, are unable to use each other as test subjects and may have to find a third person to be a test partner.

Disqualification

Both skepticism (calibrates at 160) and cynicism calibrate below 200 because they reflect negative prejudgment. In contrast, true inquiry requires an open mind and honesty devoid of intellectual vanity. Negative studies of behavioral kinesiology all calibrate below 200 (usually at 160), as do the investigators themselves.

That even famous professors can and do calibrate below 200 may seem surprising to the average person.

Thus, negative studies are a consequence of negative bias. As an example, Francis Crick's research design that led to the discovery of the double helix pattern of DNA calibrated at 440. His last research design, which was intended to prove that consciousness was just a product of neuronal activity, calibrated at only 135.

The failure of investigators who themselves, or by faulty research design, calibrate below 200 confirms the truth of the very methodology they claim to disprove. They "should" get negative results, and so they do, which paradoxically proves the accuracy of the test to detect the difference between unbiased integrity and non-integrity.

Any new discovery may upset the apple cart and be viewed as a threat to the status quo of prevailing belief systems. That a clinical science of consciousness has emerged that validates spiritual Reality is, of course, going to precipitate resistance, as it is actually a direct confrontation to the dominion of the narcissistic core of the ego itself, which is innately presumptuous and opinionated.

Below consciousness level 200, comprehension is limited by the dominance of Lower Mind, which is capable of recognizing facts but not yet able to grasp what is meant by the term "truth" (it confuses *res interna* with *res externa*) and that truth has physiological accompaniments which are different from those of falsehood. Additionally, truth is intuited as evidenced by the use of voice analysis, the study of body language, papillary response, EEG changes in the brain, fluctuations in breathing and blood pressure, galvanic skin response, dowsing, and even the Huna technique of measuring the distance that the aura radiates from the body. Some people have a very simple technique that utilizes the standing body like a pendulum (fall forward with truth and backward with falsehood).

From a more advanced contextualization, the principles that prevail are that Truth cannot be disproved by falsehood any more than light can be disproved by darkness. The nonlinear is not subject to the limitations of the linear. Truth is of a different paradigm from logic and thus is not "provable," as that which is provable calibrates only in the 400s. Consciousness research kinesiology operates at level 600, which is at the interface of the linear and the nonlinear dimensions.

CHAPTER 3

Test Results and Interpretation

The goal of this study is to generate a practical map of the energy fields of consciousness so as to delineate the range and general geography of an uncharted area of human investigation. In order to make this more easily comprehensible for the reader, the numerical designations arrived at for the various energy fields have been rounded off to comparative figures.

As we look at the Map of Consciousness (following page), it becomes clear that the calibrated levels correlate with specific processes of consciousness—emotions, perceptions or attitudes, world views and spiritual beliefs. If space permitted, the chart could be extended to include all areas of human behavior. Throughout, the research results were mutually corroborating; the more detailed and extensive the investigation, the greater was the corroboration.

MAP OF CONSCIOUSNESS®

God-view	Life-view	Level	Log	Emotion	Process
Self	Is	Enlightenment ⇧	700-1000	Ineffable	Pure Consciousness
All-Being	Perfect	Peace ⇧	600	Bliss	Illumination
One	Complete	Joy ⇧	540	Serenity	Transfiguration
Loving	Benign	Love ⇧	500	Reverence	Revelation
Wise	Meaningful	Reason ⇧	400	Understanding	Abstraction
Merciful	Harmonious	Acceptance ⇧	350	Forgiveness	Transcendence
Inspiring	Hopeful	Willingness ⇧	310	Optimism	Intention
Enabling	Satisfactory	Neutrality ⇧	250	Trust	Release

Permitting	Feasible	Courage	⇔ 200	Affirmation	Enpowerment
Indifferent	Demanding	Pride	⇒ 175	Scorn	Inflation
Vengeful	Antagonistic	Anger	⇒ 150	Hate	Aggression
Denying	Disappointing	Desire	⇒ 125	Craving	Enslavement
Punitive	Frightening	Fear	⇒ 100	Anxiety	Withdrawal
Disdainful	Tragic	Grief	⇒ 75	Regret	Despondency
Condemning	Hopeless	Apathy	⇒ 50	Despair	Abdication
Vindictive	Evil	Guilt	⇒ 30	Blame	Destruction
Despising	Miserable	Shame	⇒ 20	Humiliation	Elimination

The critical response point in the scale of consciousness calibrates at level 200, which is the level associated with Courage. All attitudes, thoughts, feelings, associations, entities, or historical figures below that level of calibration make a person go weak. Attitudes, thoughts, feelings, associations, entities, or historical figures that calibrate higher make subjects go strong. This is the balance point between weak and strong attractors, between negative and positive influence, and between truth and falsehood.

At the levels below 200, the primary impetus is survival, although at the very bottom of the scale—the zone of hopelessness and depression—even that motive is lacking. The levels of Fear and Anger are characterized by egocentric impulses, which arise from this drive for personal survival. At the level of Pride, the survival motive may expand to include the survival of others as well. As one crosses the demarcation between negative and positive influence and goes on into Courage, the well-being of others becomes increasingly important. By the 500 level, the happiness of others emerges as the essential motivating force. The high 500s are characterized by interest in spiritual awareness for both oneself and others, and by the 600s, the good of mankind and the search for enlightenment are the primary goals. From 700 to 1,000, life is dedicated to the salvation of all of humanity.

Discussion

Reflection on this map can bring about a profound expansion of one's empathy for life in its variety of expressions. If we examine what are generally held to be less "virtuous" emotional attitudes, we realize they are essentially neither good nor bad; moralistic judgments are merely a function of the viewpoint from which they emanate.

We see, for instance, that a person in Grief, which calibrates at the energy level of 75, will be in a much better condition if he rises to Anger, which calibrates at 150. Anger itself, however, is a destructive emotion and is still a low state of consciousness, but as social history shows, Apathy can imprison entire subcultures as well as individuals. If the hopeless can come to wanting something better (Desire at 125) and then use the energy of Anger at 150 to develop Pride at 175, they may then be able to take the step to Courage, which calibrates at 200, and proceed to actually ameliorate their individual or collective conditions.

Conversely, the person who has arrived at a habitual state of unconditional Love will experience anything less to be unacceptable. As one advances in the evolution of his individual consciousness, the process becomes self-perpetuating and self-correcting so that self-improvement becomes a way of life. This phenomenon can be commonly observed among members of 12-step groups who constantly work at overcoming negative attitudes such as self-pity or intolerance. People further down on the scale of consciousness may find these same attitudes acceptable and will even righteously defend them.

Throughout history, all of the world's great religions and spiritual disciplines have been concerned with techniques to ascend through these levels of consciousness. Most have also implied, or specifically stated, that to move up this ladder is an arduous task and that success depends on having a teacher (or at least teachings) to give specific instruction and inspiration to the aspirant, who might otherwise despair over his inability to achieve the goal unaided. Hopefully, our chart will help to facilitate this ultimate human endeavor.

The epistemological effect of awareness of this schema is subtle, but can be far-reaching; implications of these findings have pragmatic applications to sports, medicine, psychiatry, psychology, personal relationships, and the general quest for happiness. Contemplation of the Map of Consciousness can, for instance, transform one's understanding of causality. As perception itself evolves with one's level of consciousness, it becomes apparent that what the world calls the domain of causes is in fact the domain of effects. By taking responsibility for the consequences of their own perceptions, observers can transcend the role of victim to an understanding that "nothing out there has power over you." It is not life's events, but how one reacts to them and the attitude that one has about them, which determine whether the events have a positive or negative effect on one's life, whether they are experienced as opportunity or as stress.

Psychological stress is the net effect of a condition that you are resisting or wish to escape, but the condition does not have any power in and of itself. Nothing has the power within itself to "create" stress. The loud music that raises the blood pressure of one person can be a source of delight to another. A divorce may be traumatic if it is unwanted, or a release into freedom if it is desired.

The Map of Consciousness also casts a new light on the progress of history. A most important distinction for the purpose of this study is that between force and power. We can, for example, investigate an historical epoch, such as the end of British colonialism in India. If we calibrate the position of the British Empire at the time, which was one of self-interest and exploitation, we find that it was well below the critical level of 200 on the scale of consciousness. The motivation of Mahatma Gandhi (calibrated at 760) was very near the top of the range of normal human consciousness. Gandhi won in this struggle because his position was one of far greater power. The British Empire (calibrated at 175), represented force and, whenever force meets power, force is eventually defeated.

We may observe how throughout history, society has tried to "treat" social problems by legislative action, warfare, market manipulation, laws, and prohibitions— all manifestations of force—only to see these problems persist or recur despite the treatment. Although governments (or individuals) proceeding from positions of force are myopic, to the sensitive observer it eventually becomes obvious that conditions of social conflict will not disappear until the underlying etiology has been exposed and "healed."

The difference between treating and healing is that in the former, the context remains the same, whereas in the latter, the clinical response is elicited by a change of context so as to bring about an absolute removal of the basis of the condition rather than mere recovery from its symptoms. It is one thing to prescribe an anti-hypertensive medication for high blood pressure; it is quite another to expand the patient's context of life to the degree that he stops being angry, hostile, and repressive.

The empathy derived from contemplating this Map of Consciousness will hopefully make it a shorter step to Joy. The key to Joy is unconditional kindness to all of life, including one's own, which we refer to as compassion.[1] Without compassion, little of any significance is ever accomplished in human endeavor. We may generalize to the greater social context from individual therapies, wherein patients cannot be truly cured or fundamentally healed until they invoke the power of compassion, both for themselves and others. At that point, the healed may become a healer.

CHAPTER 4

Levels of Human Consciousness

Millions of calibrations over the years of this study have defined a range of values accurately corresponding to well-recognized sets of attitudes and emotions, localized by specific attractor energy fields, much as electromagnetic fields gather iron fillings. We have adopted the following classification of these energy fields so as to be easily comprehensible, as well as clinically and subjectively accurate.

It is very important to remember that the calibration figures do not represent an arithmetic, but a *logarithmic*, progression. Thus, the level 300 is not twice the amplitude of 150; it is 300 to the 10th power (10^{300}). Therefore, an increase of even a few points represents a major advance in power; the rate of increase in power as we move up the scale is therefore enormous.

The ways the various levels of human consciousness express themselves are profound and far-reaching; their effects are both gross and subtle. All levels below 200 are destructive of life in both the individual and society at large; in contrast, all levels above 200 are constructive expressions of power. The decisive level of 200 is the fulcrum that divides the general areas of force (or falsehood) from power (or truth).

In describing the emotional correlates of the energy fields of consciousness, it is well to remember that they are rarely manifested as pure states in an individual. A person may operate on one level in a given area of life and on quite a different level in another area of life. An individual's overall level of consciousness is the sum total effect of all these various levels.

Energy Level 20: Shame

The level of Shame is perilously proximate to death, which may be chosen out of Shame as conscious suicide or more subtly elected by failure to take steps to prolong life, as in "passive suicide." Death by avoidable accident is common. We all have some awareness of the pain of "losing face," becoming discredited, or feeling like a "nonperson." In Shame, people hang their heads and slink away, wishing they were invisible. Banishment is a traditional accompaniment of shame and, in the primitive societies from which we all originate, banishment is equivalent to death.

Early life experiences such as sexual abuse, which lead to Shame, warp the personality often for a lifetime unless these issues are resolved by therapy. Shame, as Freud determined, produces neurosis. It is destructive to emotional and psychological health and, as a consequence of low self-esteem, makes one prone to the development of physical illness. The Shame-based personality is shy, withdrawn, and introverted.

Shame is also used as a tool of cruelty, and its victims often become cruel themselves. Shamed children are cruel to animals and cruel to each other. The behavior of people whose consciousness level is only in the 20s is dangerous. They are prone to hallucinations of an accusatory nature, as well as paranoia; some become psychotic or commit bizarre crimes.

Some Shame-based individuals compensate by perfectionism and rigidity, and often become driven and intolerant. Notorious examples of this are the moral extremists who form vigilante groups, projecting their own unconscious shame onto others whom they then feel justified in righteously attacking or killing. Serial killers have often acted out of sexual moralism, with the justification of punishing so-called "bad" women.

Because it pulls down the whole level of one's personality, Shame results in a vulnerability to the other negative emotions, and, therefore, often produces false pride, anger, and guilt.

Energy Level 30: Guilt

Guilt, so commonly used in our society to manipulate and punish, manifests itself in a variety of expressions, such as remorse, self-recrimination, masochism, and the whole gamut of symptoms of victimhood. Unconscious Guilt results in psychosomatic disease, accident-proneness, and suicidal behaviors. Many people struggle with Guilt their entire lives, while others desperately attempt escape by amorally denying Guilt altogether.

Guilt-domination results in a preoccupation with "sin," an unforgiving emotional attitude frequently exploited by religious demagogues, who use it for coercion and control. Such "sin-and-salvation" merchants, obsessed with punishment, are likely either acting out their own guilt, or projecting it on to others.

Subcultures displaying the aberration of self-flagellation often manifest other endemic forms of cruelty, such as the public, ritual killing of humans or animals. Guilt provokes rage, and killing frequently is its expression. Capital punishment is an example of how killing gratifies a Guilt-ridden populace. Our unforgiving

American society, for instance, pillories its victims in the press and metes out punishments that have never been demonstrated to have any deterrent or corrective effect.

Energy Level 50: Apathy

This level is characterized by poverty, despair, and hopelessness. The world and the future look bleak; pathos is the theme of life. Apathy is a state of helplessness; its victims, needy in every way, lack not only resources but also the energy to avail themselves of what resources may be available. Unless external energy is supplied by caregivers, death through passive suicide can result. Without the will to live, the hopeless stare blankly, unresponsive to stimuli, until their eyes stop tracking and there is not even enough energy left to swallow proffered food.

This is the level of the homeless and the derelicts of society; it is also the fate of many of the aged and others who become isolated by chronic or progressive diseases. The apathetic are dependent; people in Apathy are "heavy" and are felt to be a burden by those around them.

Too often, society lacks sufficient motivation to be of any real help to cultures as well as individuals at this level, who are seen as drains of resources. This is the level of the streets of Calcutta, where only the saintly such as Mother Teresa and her followers dare to tread. Apathy is the level of the abandonment of hope, and few have the courage to really look it in the face.

Energy Level 75: Grief

This is the level of sadness, loss, and despondency.

Most humans have experienced it for periods of time, but those who remain at this level live a life of constant regret and depression. This is the level of chronic mourning, bereavement, and remorse about the past; it is also the level of habitual losers and those chronic gamblers who accept failure as part of their lifestyle, often resulting in loss of jobs, friends, family, and opportunity, as well as money and health.

Major losses in early life make one later vulnerable to passive acceptance of grief, as though sorrow were the price of life. In Grief, one sees sadness everywhere: the sadness of little children, the sadness of world conditions, the sadness of life itself. This level colors one's entire vision of existence (Part of the syndrome of loss is the notion of the irreplaceability of what has been lost or that which it symbolized. There is a generalization from the particular so that the loss of a loved one is equated with the loss of love itself. At this level, such emotional losses may trigger a serious depression or death.

Although Grief is the cemetery of life, it still has more energy to it than Apathy does. Thus, when a traumatized, apathetic patient begins to cry, we know they are getting better. Once they start to cry, they will begin to eat again.

Energy Level 100: Fear
At the level of 100, there is a lot more life energy available; fear of danger is actually healthy. Fear runs much of the world, spurring on endless activity. Fear of enemies, of old age or death, of rejection, and a multitude of social fears are basic motivators in most

people's lives.

From the viewpoint of this level, the world looks hazardous, full of traps and threats. Fear is the favored official tool for control by oppressive totalitarian agencies and regimes, and insecurity is the stock-in-trade of major manipulators of the marketplace. The media and advertising play to Fear to increase market share.

The proliferation of fears is as limitless as the human imagination; once Fear becomes one's focus, the endless fearful events of the world feed it. Fear becomes obsessive and may take any form. Fear of loss of relationship leads to jealousy and a chronically high stress level. Fearful thinking can balloon into paranoia or generate neurotic defensive structures and, because it is contagious, become a dominant social trend.

Fear limits growth of the personality and leads to inhibition. Because it takes energy to rise above Fear, the oppressed are unable to reach a higher level unaided. Thus, the fearful seek strong leaders who appear to have conquered their fear to lead them out of their slavery.

Energy Level 125: Desire

There is yet more energy available at this level; Desire motivates vast areas of human activity, including the economy. Advertisers play on our Desire to program us with needs linked to instinctual drives. Desire moves us to expend great effort to achieve goals or obtain rewards. The desire for money, prestige, or power runs the lives of many of those who have risen above Fear as their limiting, predominant life motif.

Desire is also the level of addiction, wherein desire

becomes a craving more important than life itself.
The victims of Desire may actually be unaware of the
basis of their motives. Some people become addicted
to the desire for attention and drive others away by
their constant demands. The desire for sexual
approval has produced entire cosmetics, fashion, and
movie industries.

HUNGRY GHOSTS

Desire has to do with accumulation and greed. But
Desire is insatiable because it is an ongoing energy
field, so that satisfaction of one desire is merely
replaced by unsatisfied desire for something else.
Multimillionaires remain obsessed with acquiring more
and more money.

Desire, however, is a much higher state than Apathy
or Grief. In order to "get," you have to first have the
energy to "want." Television has had a major influence
on many oppressed people, because it inculcates wants
and energizes their desires to the degree that they
move out of Apathy and begin to seek a better life.
Want can start people on the road to achievement.
Desire can, therefore, become a springboard to higher
levels of consciousness.

Energy Level 150: Anger

Although Anger may lead to homicide and war, as an
energy level within itself it is much further removed
from death than those below it. Anger can lead to
either constructive or destructive action. As people
move out of Apathy and Grief to overcome Fear as a
way of life, they begin to want; Desire leads to frustration, which in turn leads to Anger. Thus, Anger can
be a fulcrum by which the oppressed are eventually

catapulted to freedom. Anger over social injustice, victimization, and inequality has created great movements that led to major changes in the structure of society.

But Anger expresses itself most often as resentment and revenge and is, therefore, volatile and dangerous. Anger as a lifestyle is exemplified by irritable, explosive people who are oversensitive to slights and become "injustice collectors," quarrelsome, belligerent, or litigious.

Since Anger stems from frustrated want, it is based on the energy field below it. Frustration results from exaggerating the importance of desires. The angry person may, like a frustrated infant, go into a rage. Anger leads easily to hatred, which has an erosive effect on all areas of a person's life.

Energy Level 175: Pride

Pride, which calibrates at 175, has enough energy to run the United States Marine Corps. It is the level aspired to by the majority of our kind today. People feel positive as they reach this level, in contrast to the lower energy fields. This rise in self-esteem is a balm to all the pain experienced at lower levels of consciousness. Pride looks good and knows it; it struts its stuff in the parade of life. Pride is at a far enough removal from Shame, Guilt, or Fear that to rise, for instance, out of the despair of the ghetto to the pride of being a Marine is an enormous jump. Pride as such generally has a good reputation and is socially encouraged, yet as we see from the chart of the levels of consciousness, it is sufficiently negative to remain below the critical level of 200. This is why Pride feels good only in contrast to the lower levels.

The problem, as we all know, is that "Pride goeth before a fall." Pride is defensive and vulnerable because it is dependent upon external conditions, without which it can suddenly revert to a lower level. The inflated ego is vulnerable to attack. Pride remains weak because it can be knocked off its pedestal back into Shame, which is the threat that fires the fear of loss of Pride.

Pride is divisive and gives rise to factionalism; the consequences are costly. Man has habitually died for Pride; armies still regularly slaughter each other for that aspect of Pride called nationalism. Religious wars, political terrorism and zealotry, the ghastly history of the Middle East and Central Europe, are all the price of Pride, which all of society pays.

The downside of Pride, therefore, is arrogance and denial. These characteristics block growth; in Pride, recovery from addictions is impossible because emotional problems or character defects are denied. The whole problem of denial is one of Pride. Thus Pride is a very sizable block to the acquisition of real power, which displaces Pride with true stature and prestige.

Energy Level 200: Courage

At the 200 level, power really first appears. When we test subjects at all the energy levels below 200, we find, as can be readily verified, that they all go weak. Everyone goes strong in response to the life-supportive fields above 200. This is the critical level that distinguishes the positive and negative influences of life. At the level of Courage, an attainment of true power occurs; therefore, it is also the level of empowerment. This is the zone of exploration, accomplishment, fortitude, and determination. At the lower levels, the world is seen as hopeless, sad, frightening, or frustrating; but at the level of Courage, life is seen to be exciting, challenging, and stimulating.

Courage implies the willingness to try new things and deal with the vicissitudes of life. At this level of empowerment, one is able to cope with and effectively handle the opportunities of life. At 200, for instance, there is the energy to learn new job skills. Growth and education become attainable goals. There is the capacity to face fears or character defects and to grow despite them; anxiety also does not cripple endeavor as it would at the lower levels of evolution. Obstacles that defeat people whose consciousness is below 200 act as stimulants to those who have evolved into the first level of true power.

People at this level put back into the world as much energy as they take; at lower levels, populations as well as individuals drain energy from society without reciprocating. Because accomplishments result in positive feedback, self-reward and esteem become progressively self-reinforcing. This is where productivity begins. The collective level of consciousness of mankind remained at 190 for many centuries and, curiously, only jumped to its current level of 204 within the last decade.

Energy Level 250: Neutrality

Energy becomes very positive as we get to the level that we have termed Neutral, because it is epitomized by release from the positionality that typifies lower levels.

Below 250, consciousness tends to see dichotomies and to take on rigid positions, an impediment in a world that is complex and multi-factorial rather than black and white.

Taking such positions creates polarization, and polarization in turn creates opposition and division. As in the martial arts, a rigid position becomes a point of vulnerability; that which does not bend is liable to break. Rising above barriers or oppositions that dissipate one's energies, the Neutral condition allows for flexibility and nonjudgmental, realistic appraisal of problems. To be Neutral means to be relatively unattached to outcomes; not getting one's way is no longer experienced as defeating, frightening, or frustrating.

At the Neutral level, a person can say, "Well, if I don't get this job, then I'll get another." This is the beginning of inner confidence; sensing one's power, one is therefore not easily intimidated. One is not driven to prove anything. The expectation that life, with its ups and downs, will be basically okay if one can roll with the punches is a typical 250-level attitude.

People of Neutrality have a sense of well-being; the mark of this level is a confident capability to live in the world. This is, therefore, experientially a level of safety. People at this level are easy to get along with, safe to be around and associate with, because they are not interested in conflict, competition, or guilt. They are comfortable and basically undisturbed emotionally. This attitude is nonjudgmental and does not lead to any need to control other people's behaviors. Correspondingly, because Neutral people value freedom, they are hard to control.

Energy Level 310: <u>Willingness</u>

This very positive level of energy may be seen as the gateway to the higher levels. Whereas for instance, jobs are done adequately at the Neutral level, at the level of Willingness, work is done well and success in all endeavors is common. Growth is rapid; these are people chosen for advancement. Willingness implies that one has overcome inner resistance to life and is committed to participation. Below the 200 calibration level, people tend to be close-minded, but by level 310, a great opening occurs. At this level, people become genuinely friendly, and social and economic success seem to follow automatically. The Willing are not really troubled by unemployment, for they will take any job when they have to, or create a career or self-employ- ment for themselves. They do not feel demeaned by service jobs or by starting at the bottom. They are naturally helpful to others and contribute to the good of society. They are also willing to face inner issues and do not have major learning blocks.

At this level, self-esteem is innately high and is reinforced by positive feedback from society in the forms of recognition, appreciation, and reward. Willingness is sympathetic and responsive to the needs of others. Willing people are builders of, and contribu- tors to, society. With their capacity to bounce back from adversity and learn from experience, they tend to become self-correcting. Having let go of Pride, they are willing to look at their own defects and learn from others. At the level of Willingness, people become excellent students. They are easily teachable and represent a considerable source of power for society.

Energy Level 350: Acceptance

At this level of awareness, a major transformation takes place, with the understanding that one is oneself the source and creator of the experience of one's life. Taking such responsibility is distinctive of this degree of evolution, characterized by the capacity to live harmoniously with the forces of life.

All people at levels below 200 tend to be powerless and see themselves as victims, at the mercy of life. This stems from a belief that the source of one's happiness or the cause of one's problems is "out there." An enormous jump—taking back one's own power—is completed at this level, with the realization that the source of happiness is within oneself. At this more evolved stage, nothing so-called "out there" has the capacity to make one happy, and love is not something that is given or taken away by another, but is created from within.

Acceptance is not to be confused with passivity, which is a symptom of apathy. This form of Acceptance allows engagement in life on life's own terms, without trying to make it conform to an agenda. With Acceptance, there is emotional calm and perception is widened as denial is transcended. One now sees things without distortion or misinterpretation; the context of experience is expanded so that one is capable of "seeing the whole picture." Acceptance has to do essentially with balance, proportion, and appropriateness.

The individual at the level of Acceptance is not interested in determining right or wrong, but instead is dedicated to resolving issues and finding out what to do about problems. Tough jobs do not cause discomfort or dismay. Long-term goals take precedence over short-term ones; self-discipline and mastery are prominent.

At the level of Acceptance, we are not polarized by conflict or opposition; we see that other people have the same rights as we do, and we honor equality. While lower levels are characterized by rigidity, at this level, social plurality begins to emerge as a form of resolution of problems. Therefore, this level is free of discrimination or intolerance; there is the awareness that equality does not preclude diversity. Acceptance includes rather than rejects.

Energy Level 400: Reason

Intelligence and rationality rise to the forefront when the emotionalism of the lower levels is transcended. Reason is capable of handling large, complex amounts of data; making rapid, correct decisions; understanding the intricacies of relationships, gradations, and fine distinctions; and expert manipulation of symbols as abstract concepts, which becomes increasingly important. This is the level of science, medicine, and of generally increased capability for conceptualization and comprehension. Knowledge and education are sought as capital. Understanding and information are the main tools of accomplishment, which is the hallmark of the 400 level. This is the level of Nobel Prize winners, great statesmen, and Supreme Court justices. Einstein, Freud, and many of the other great thinkers of history also calibrate here. The authors of the *Great Books of the Western World* calibrate here.

The shortcomings of this level are the failure to

clearly distinguish the difference between symbols and what they represent, and confusion between the objective and subjective worlds that limits the understanding of causality. At this level, it is easy to lose sight of the forest for the trees, to become infatuated with concepts and theories, ending up in intellectualism and missing the essential point. Intellectualizing can become an end in itself. Reason is limited in that it does not afford the capacity for the discernment of essence or of the critical point of a complex issue. And it generally disregards context.

Reason does not of itself provide a guide to truth. It produces massive amounts of information and documentation, but lacks the capability to resolve discrepancies in data and conclusions. All philosophic arguments sound convincing on their own. Although Reason is highly effective in a technical world where the methodologies of logic dominate, Reason itself, paradoxically, is the major block to reaching higher levels of consciousness. Transcending this level is relatively uncommon—by only 4.0 percent of the world's population.

Energy Level 500: Love

Love as depicted in the mass media is not what this level implies. On the contrary, what the world generally refers to as love is an intense emotionality combining physical attraction, possessiveness, control, addiction, eroticism, and novelty. It is usually evanescent and fluctuating, waxing and waning with varying conditions. When frustrated, this emotion often reveals an underlying anger and dependency that it had masked.

That love can turn to hate is a common concept, but what is being spoken about rather than love is an addictive sentimentality and attachment. Hate stems from Pride, not Love. There probably never was actual Love in such a relationship.

The 500 level is characterized by the development of a Love that is unconditional, unchanging, and permanent. It does not fluctuate because its source within the person who loves is not dependent on external conditions. Loving is a state of being. It is a way of relating to the world that is forgiving, nurturing, and supportive. Love is not intellectual and does not proceed from the mind. Love emanates from the heart. It has the capacity to lift others and accomplish great feats because of its purity of motive.

As this level of development, the capacity to discern essence becomes predominant; the core of an issue becomes the center of focus. As reason is bypassed, there arises the capacity for instantaneous recognition of the totality of a problem and a major expansion of context, especially regarding time and process. Reason deals only with particulars, whereas Love deals with wholes. This ability, often ascribed to intuition, is the capacity for instantaneous understanding without resorting to sequential symbol processing. This apparently abstract phenomenon is, in fact, quite concrete; it is accompanied by a measurable release of endorphins in the brain.

Love takes no position and thus is global, rising above the separation of positionality. It is then possible to be "one with another," as there are no longer any barriers. Love is therefore inclusive and expands the

sense of self progressively. Love focuses on the good-
ness of life in all its expressions and augments that
which is positive. It dissolves negativity by recontextualizing it rather than by attacking it.

This is the level of true happiness, but although the
world is fascinated with the subject of Love, and all
viable religions calibrate at 500 or over, it is interesting
to note that only 4.0 percent of the world's population
ever reaches this level of the evolution of consciousness. Only 0.4 percent ever reaches the level of
unconditional love at 540.

Energy Level 540: Joy

As Love becomes more and more unconditional,
it begins to be experienced as an inner Joy. This is
not the sudden joy of a pleasurable turn of events; it
is a constant accompaniment to all activities. Joy arises
from within each moment of existence, rather than
from any external source. 540 is also the level of healing and of spiritually based self-help groups.

From level 540 and up is the domain of saints,
spiritual healers, and advanced spiritual students.
Characteristic of this energy field is the capacity for
enormous patience and the persistence of a positive
attitude in the face of prolonged adversity. The hallmark of this state is compassion. People who have
attained this level have a notable effect on others. They
are capable of a prolonged, open visual gaze, which
induces a state of love and peace.

At the high 500s, the world one sees is illuminated
by the exquisite beauty and perfection of creation.
Everything happens effortlessly, by synchronicity, and

the world and everything in it is seen to be an expression of love and Divinity. Individual will merges into Divine will. A Presence is felt whose power facilitates phenomena outside conventional expectations of reality, termed miraculous by the ordinary observer. These phenomena represent the power of the energy field, not that of the individual.

One's sense of responsibility for others at this level is of a different quality from that shown at the lower levels. There is a desire to use one's state of consciousness for the benefit of life itself rather than for particular individuals. This capacity to love many people simultaneously is accompanied by the discovery that the more one loves, the more one can love.

Near-death experiences, characteristically transformative in their effect, have frequently allowed people to experience the energy level between 540 and 600.

Energy Level 600: Peace
This energy field is associated with the experience designated by such terms as transcendence, self-realization, and God-consciousness. It is extremely rare. When this state is reached, the distinction between subject and object disappears, and there is no specific focal point of perception. Not uncommonly, individuals at this level remove themselves from the world, as the state of bliss that ensues precludes ordinary activity. Some become spiritual teachers; others work anonymously for the betterment of mankind. A few become great geniuses in their respective fields and make major contributions to society. These people are saintly and may eventually be designated officially as saints,

although at this level, formal religion is commonly transcended, to be replaced by the pure spirituality out of which all religion originates.

Perception at the level of 600 and above is sometimes reported as occurring in slow motion, suspended in time and space—though nothing is stationary; all is alive and radiant. Although this world is the same world as the one seen by others, it has become continuously flowing, evolving in an exquisitely coordinated evolutionary dance in which significance and source are overwhelming. This awesome revelation takes place non-rationally, so that there is an infinite silence in the mind, which has stopped conceptualizing. That which is witnessing and that which is witnessed take on the same identity; the observer dissolves into the landscape and becomes equally the observed. Everything is connected to everything else by a Presence whose power is infinite, exquisitely gentle, yet rock-solid.

Great works of art, music, and architecture that calibrate between 600 and 700 can transport us temporarily to higher levels of consciousness and are universally recognized as inspirational and timeless.

Energy Levels 700-1,000: Enlightenment

This is the level of the Great Ones of history who originated the spiritual patterns that multitudes have followed throughout the ages. All are associated with Divinity, with which they are often identified. This is the level of powerful inspiration; these beings set in place attractor energy fields that influence all of mankind down through the ages. At this level, there is no longer the experience of an individual personal self as separate from others; rather, there is an identification of Self with Consciousness and Divinity. The Unmanifest is experienced as Self beyond mind. This transcendence of the ego also serves by example to teach others how it can eventually be accomplished. This is the peak of the evolution of consciousness in the human realm.

Great teachings uplift the masses and raise the level of awareness of all of humanity. To have such vision is called grace, and the gift it brings is infinite peace, described as ineffable, beyond words.[1] At this level of realization, the sense of one's existence transcends all time and all individuality. There is no longer any identification with the physical body as "me," and therefore, its fate is of no concern. The body is seen as merely a tool of consciousness through the intervention of mind, its prime value that of communication. The self merges back into the Self. This is the level of nonduality, or complete Oneness. There is no localization of consciousness; awareness is everywhere equally present.[2]

Great works of art depicting individuals who have reached the level of Enlightenment characteristically show the teacher with a specific hand position, called a mudra, wherein the palm of the hand radiates benediction. This is the act of the transmission of this energy field to the consciousness of mankind. This level of Divine Grace calibrates up to 1,000, the highest level attained by any persons who have lived in recorded history—to wit, the Great Avatars for whom the title "Lord" is appropriate: Lord Krishna, Lord Buddha, and Lord Jesus Christ.

CHAPTER 5

Social Distribution of Consciousness Levels

General Description

A graphic representation of the distribution of the respective energy levels among the world's population would resemble the shape of a pagoda, in that 85 percent of the human race calibrates below the critical level of 200, while the overall average level of human consciousness today is approximately 204.[1] The power of the relatively few individuals near the top counterbalances the energy of the masses toward the bottom to achieve this overall average. Only 8.0 percent of the world's population operates at the consciousness level of the 400s, only 4.0 percent of the world's population calibrates at an energy field of 500 and over, and a level of consciousness calibrating at 600 and over is reached by only one in many millions.

At first glance, these figures may seem improbable, but if we examine world conditions, we will quickly be reminded that the populations of whole subcontinents live at a bare subsistence level. Famine and disease are commonplace, frequently accompanied by political oppression and paucity of social resources. Many of such people live in a state of hopelessness calibrating at the level of Apathy, in resignation to their abject poverty. We must also realize that much of the remainder of the world's population—civilized as well as primitive—lives primarily in Fear; the majority of humans spend their lives in a quest for one form of security or another. Those whose lifestyles transcend the imperative of survival so as to allow discretionary options then become grist for the Desire-driven world economic mill, and success in attaining these desires leads at best to Pride.

Any meaningful human satisfaction cannot even commence until about the level of 250, where some degree of self-confidence begins to emerge as the basis for positive life experiences in the evolution of consciousness.

Cultural Correlations

The energy fields below 200 are most common in extremely primitive conditions where people eke out bare subsistence. Clothing is sparse, illiteracy is the rule, infant mortality is high, disease and malnutrition are widespread, and there is a vacuum of social power. Skills are rudimentary and center around fuel and food gathering and shelter preparation, and there is total dependence on the vagaries of the immediate environment. This is the Stone Age tribal cultural level, little more than animal existence.

Populations characterized by the low 200s are typified by unskilled labor, rudimentary trade, and the building of simple artifacts, such as dugout canoes and temporary housing. Mobility begins to express itself in the nomadic lifestyle and, in populations that average a somewhat higher consciousness, agriculture first appears and barter evolves into the use of token currency.

The mid-200s are associated with semi-skilled labor. Simple but life-sustaining housing and food economy become dependably available; clothing is adequate, and elementary education begins.

The high 200s are represented by skilled labor,

blue-collar workers, tradesmen, retail commerce, and industries. At lower levels, for example, fishing is an individual or a tribal activity, but above the mid-200s, it becomes an industry.

At the level of 300, we find technicians, skilled and advanced craftsmen, managers, and a more sophisticated business structure. Completion of secondary education becomes customary. There is an interest in style, sport and public entertainment; TV is the great pastime at this level.

In the mid-300s, we find upper management, artisans, and educators with an informed awareness of public events and a worldview that extends beyond the tribe, neighborhood, or city to the nation at large and its welfare. Social dialogue becomes a meaningful matter of interest. Survival has been assured by the acquisition of skills and information adequate to function as a civilized society. There is social mobility and flexibility, and resources that enable a limited amount of travel and other stimulating recreation.

The 400s are the level of the awakening of the intellect, the locus of true literacy, higher education, the professional class, executives, and scientists. The home, devoid of reading materials at the lower levels, now exhibits magazines, periodicals, and full bookcases. There is an interest in educational broadcast channels on TV, and a more sophisticated political awareness. Great communication adeptness, intellectual preoccupation, and artistic creativity are common. Recreational activities take the form of chess, travel, theater, and concerts. Civic enterprises intended to enhance the social milieu receive serious attention.

Supreme Court justices, presidents, statesmen, inventors, and leaders of industry occupy this general range.

Because education is the underpinning of this level,
individuals tend to gather in metropolitan areas where
they have access to sources of information and
instruction, such as the great universities. Some aspire
to faculty status, while others become lawyers or
members of other professional classes. The welfare of
one's fellow man is a common concern, though not yet
a driving force. The high 400s are associated with leaders
in their respective fields, and with high social prestige,
accomplishment, and corresponding social trappings.
Both Einstein and Freud calibrated at 499. But while
the 400s are the level of universities and doctorates,
they are also the source of the limited and limiting
Newtonian visions of the universe and of the Cartesian
split between mind and body. Interestingly, both
Newton and Descartes calibrated at 499.

Just as the level 200 demarcates a critical change of
consciousness, 500 is a point at which awareness
makes another great leap. Although survival of the
individual is still important, the motivation of Love
begins to color all activities, and creativity comes into
full expression, accompanied by commitment, dedication, and expressions of charisma. Here, excellence is
common in every field of human endeavor, from sport
to scientific investigation. Altruism becomes a motivating factor, along with dedication to principles.
Leadership is accepted rather than sought. From this
level emerge great music, art, and architecture, and the
capacity to uplift others by one's mere presence.

In the upper 500s are found the inspirational leaders

who set an example for the rest of society and, in their respective fields, create new paradigms with far-reaching implications for all of mankind. Although well aware themselves that they still have defects and limitations, people on this level are often seen by the general public as out of the ordinary and may be recognized with emblems of distinction. Many people in the mid-500s begin to have spiritual experiences of profound import and become immersed in spiritual pursuit. Some astonish their friends and families with sudden breakthroughs into new, subjective contexts of reality. Consciousness at this level can be described as visionary and may focus on uplifting society as a whole. From this level, a few make the great leap to the region that calibrates at 600. At this point, an individual's life may become legendary. The signature of the 600s is compassion, which pervades all motivation and activity.

Progression of Consciousness

Although the levels we have described span a great variation, it is not common for individuals to move from one level to another during one lifetime. The energy field that is calibrated for an individual at birth only increases, on the average, by about five points. That an individual's level of consciousness is already in effect at birth is a sobering fact with profound implications. And consciousness itself, in its expression as human civilization, evolves slowly indeed, through numerous generations.

The majority of people utilize their life experiences to elaborate and express the variations of their native energy field; it is the rare individual who manages to move beyond it, although many people make considerable internal improvements. The reason for this is more easily understandable when we see that what defines one's level is motivation. Motivation proceeds from meaning, and meaning, in turn, is an expression of context. Thus, achievement is bounded by context, which, when correspondingly aligned with motivation, determines the individual's relative power.

The average advance of five points in a lifetime is, of course, a statistical figure, produced by, among other things, the fact that people's cumulative life choices not uncommonly result in a net lowering of their level of consciousness. As will be enumerated in detail later (see Chapter 23), the influence of a very few individuals of advanced consciousness counterbalances whole populations at the lower levels. But, conversely, the extreme negativity of a few individuals can sway entire cultures and produce a global drag on the general level of consciousness, as history illustrates all too well. Kinesiologic testing indicates that a mere 2.6 percent of the human population, identifiable by an abnormal kinesiologic polarity (they test strong to negative attractors and weak to positive attractors), accounts for 72 percent of society's problems.

Nonetheless, it is possible for isolated individuals to make sudden positive jumps, even of hundreds of points. If one can truly escape the egocentric entrainment of the sub-200 attractor fields, consciously choosing a friendly, earnest, kind, and forgiving approach to life, and eventually making charity toward others one's primary focus, higher levels can certainly be attained, at least in theory. In practice, great will is required.

Thus, although it is not ordinary to move out of one energy field into another during one lifetime, the opportunity still exists. It remains for motivation to activate that potential; without the exercise of choice, no progression will occur. It is well to re-emphasize that the progression of the calibrated power levels is logarithmic; thus, individual choice can have a mighty effect. The difference in power level, for instance, between 361.0 and 361.1 is very significant and capable of transforming both one's life and one's effect on the world at large.

CHAPTER 6

New Horizons in Research

Our concern thus far has been primarily to elucidate the structure and the anatomy of consciousness, with some reference to the mechanisms of force and power. But ours is in no sense a purely theoretical subject. The unique nature of the research method described herein allows exploration of hitherto inaccessible areas of potential knowledge. It is as applicable to the most prosaic practical questions as to the most advanced theoretical explorations. Let us investigate a few general examples.

Social Problems

Drug and alcohol addiction is a crucial social concern that feeds the parallel problems of crime, poverty, and welfare. Addiction has proved an intractable social and clinical problem, thus far not understood beyond the most basic description. By the term "addiction," we mean clinical addiction in the classical sense of continued dependence on alcohol or drugs despite serious consequences, a condition exceeding the capacity of the addicted person to discontinue use of the substance unaided, because the will itself has been rendered ineffective. But what is the essential nature of addiction, and to what is the addict really addicted?

The common belief is that it is the addictive substance itself to which the victim has become addicted, because of that substance's power to create a "high" state of euphoria. But if we reexamine the nature of addiction through the methodology described, a different formulation of the process emerges. Alcohol or drugs do not, in and of themselves, have the power to create a "high" at all; they calibrate at only 100 (same as the level of vegetables). The so-called "high" that the drug or alcohol user experiences, however, can calibrate from 350 to 600. The actual effect of drugs is merely to suppress the lower energy fields, thereby allowing the user to experience exclusively only the higher ones. It is as though a filter screened out all the lower tones coming from an orchestra so that all that could be heard were the high notes. The suppression of the low notes does not create the high ones; it merely reveals their presence.

Within the levels of consciousness, the higher frequencies are extremely powerful, and few people routinely experience these as pure states because they are masked by the lower energy fields of anxiety, fear, anger, resentment, and so on. Rarely does the average person get to experience, for instance, love without fear, or pure joy, much less ecstasy. But these higher states are so powerful that once experienced, they are never forgotten, and are sought ever after.

It is to this experience of higher states that people become addicted.[1] A good illustration is presented in the classic movie, *Lost Horizon*. Shangri-La (the movie's metaphor for unconditional love and beauty) calibrates at 600. Once experienced, it reprograms the experiencer so that he is never content again with ordinary consciousness. The hero of the movie discovers this fact when he is unable to find happiness again in the ordinary world after returning from Shangri-La. He then gives up everything in order to seek out and return to that state of consciousness, spending years in a struggle, which almost costs him his life, to regain and find Shangri-La again.

This same reprogramming process occurs in people who have reached high states of consciousness by other means, such as the experience of Samadhi through meditation, or near-death experiences. Such individuals are frequently observed to have changed forever. It is not uncommon for them to leave all that the material world represents and become seekers after truth; many who had transcendent experiences with LSD in the 1960s did that very same thing. Such higher states are also attained through the experiences of love and religion, classical music or art, or through the practice of spiritual disciplines.

The high state that people seek, by whatever means, is in fact the experience field of their own consciousness (Self). If they are spiritually unsophisticated and lack a context with which to comprehend the experience, they believe it is created from something "out there" (such as a guru, music, drugs, lover, and so forth). All that has actually happened is that, under special circumstances, they have experienced their own inner reality. The majority of people are so divorced from their own states of pure consciousness that they do not recognize them when they experience them, because they identify with their lower ego states. A negative self-image blots out the joyous brilliance that is the true essence of their identities, which therefore goes unrecognized. That this joyous, peaceful, fulfilling state is in reality one's own inner essence has been the basic tenet of every great spiritual teacher (for example, "the kingdom of God is within you").[2]

A "high" is any state of consciousness above one's customary level of awareness. Therefore, to a person who lives in Fear, moving up to Courage is a "high." To people who live in hopeless Apathy, Anger is a "high" (for example, rioters in third-world ghettoes). Fear at least feels better than Despair, and Pride feels far better than Fear. Acceptance is much more comfortable than Courage; and Love makes any lower state seem comparatively unattractive. While Joy surpasses all lesser human emotions, Ecstasy is a rarely felt emotion in a class by itself. The most sublime experience of all is the state of Infinite Peace at level 600, so exquisite that it belies all attempts at description.

The higher the level of these states, the greater its power to reprogram the subject's entire life. Not uncommonly, just one instant in a very high state can completely change a person's orientation to life, as well as his goals and values. It can be said that the individual who was, is no more, and a new person is born out of the experience. Through hard-won progress on a dedicated spiritual path, this is the very mechanism of spiritual evolution.

The permanent high-state experience, which may be legitimately attained only through a lifetime of dedicated inner work, can be reached temporarily by artificial means. But the balance of nature dictates that to artificially acquire that state without having earned it creates a debt, and the negative imbalance results in negative consequences. The cost of such stolen pleasure is the desperation of addiction, and finally, both the addict and society pay a price.

Ours is a society that idealizes the pleasureless (hard work, stoicism, self-sacrifice, restraint) and tends to condemn pleasure in most of its simpler forms, frequently even declaring them to be illegal. (Politicians, whether secular or eccleslastic, understand this phenomenon well. A ploy of local politicians to gain headlines is the public announcement of intents to prohibit pleasures in the prisons, to deny the inmates tobacco or TV or magazines.)[3] In our society, unfulfilled promises and enticement are legitimized, but satisfaction is denied. Commercialized sexual allure, for instance, is used to sell many products endlessly, but the enjoyment of actual commercial sex is forbidden as immoral.

Historically, all ruling classes have achieved status and wealth by controlling society through some form of puritanical ethic. The harder the underlings work, and the more meager their pleasures, the richer the ruling system will be, whether it be a theocracy, aristocracy, oligarchy, or corporate industrial barony. Such power is built upon the forfeited pleasure of workers. Experientially, as we have seen, pleasure is merely high energy. The energies of the masses have been co-opted over the centuries to produce for the over-classes the very wealth of pleasures denied the under-classes.

In truth, the pleasure of life energy is mankind's best capital; robbing man of this has resulted in the wide division between the "haves" and the multitudes of "have-nots." What working classes envy in the lives of upper classes are their pleasures, from the pleasures of exercising power in its varied forms to the beautiful trophies of self-indulgence. The realization that the pleasures being denied oneself are being enjoyed by others begets the outrage of revolution or, sublimated, the repression of restrictive laws against the pleasures of one's peers.

The moral code thus functions as a rationalized exploitation of the life energy of the masses, through a calculated distortion of values. The illusion proffered is that the more hellish one's life, the more heavenly will be one's reward. This distorted coupling of pleasure with suffering has produced a morally perverse social milieu, in which pain becomes associated with pleasure. In this atmosphere, the extreme alternation of suffering and euphoria that typifies addiction becomes at least provisionally tenable in a deadly antisocial game of winning and losing the forbidden high.

From the same life view arises society's current method of "treating the problem" by playing the other half of the game: denying the substance of abuse. By doing so, we have created a marketplace that is so highly lucrative and easily entered that a whole criminal industry flourishes as a result, corrupting life on multiple levels. The arrest of a drug kingpin, for instance, has no effect at all on the drug problem overall; before he is even jailed, he will have already been replaced by a new one. For example, at the demise of the South American drug lord Pablo Escobar, he was instantly replaced by three new kingpins, so the hydra now had three heads instead of one.[4]

Society's drug problem requires a social approach calibrating at 350, and our current anti-drug program calibrates at only 150. Therefore, it is ineffective, and the money spent on it is wasted.

Industrial and Scientific Research

The diagnostic method we have described quickly tracks fruitful areas for research and development in science and industry. Historical examples illustrate how the use of this method can save years of effort and millions of dollars.

Materials Research

Thomas Edison tested over 1,600 substances before he arrived at tungsten as the most suitable element to be used for his historic development of the incandescent lightbulb.[5] An easier way to detect the best material was simply to divide the possible alternatives into two groups and ask, "The material is in this group." (Y/N?) After that determination, the group is again subdivided, and so on. By this method, an answer can be derived in a matter of exactly three minutes rather than years.

Product Development

RJR Nabisco Holdings Corporation spent approximately $350 million to research and produce a smokeless cigarette,[6] on the mistaken assumption that smoking is primarily an oral habit. (In fact, it has been discovered clinically that when people go blind, they tend to stop smoking. Smoking has multiple bases, of which oral gratification is only one, and even minor.)[7] A kinesiologic test of the market viability of any potential product, including the one just mentioned, can arrive at clear conclusions regarding public acceptance and feasibili-

ty of marketing in less than a minute. Product accept-
ability and profitability can be ascertained very accurately if questions are phrased with precision and all
contingencies are investigated, including timing, mar-
kets, advertising, and subpopulations to be addressed.

Scientific Inquiry

Science provides a field of kinesiologic exploration
that offers a group of inquirers excitement eclipsing
any parlor game. (It is also fascinating for a group to
compare what they have discovered with the discoveries of other groups using the same method.) In a more
general application, avenues for fruitful research can be
identified quickly, and it will be discovered that often
the most valuable insights to be obtained have to do
with the range and dimension of the research. Because
this method bypasses limitations of context, one of its
most valuable uses is as a check on the process itself;
that is, whether or not it is a correct direction to take.
We may thus confirm that the basic premises from
which inquiries originate have validity.

For instance, our current search for life elsewhere
in the universe takes the form of broadcasting into
space the mathematical symbol π. Implicit herein is the
assumption that no civilization could develop radio
reception unless it could understand that mathematical
concept. But it is so enormously presumptuous to
assume that life elsewhere is even three-dimensional or
detectable by human senses at all, let alone be composed of discrete life units that solve problems by use
of an intellect and employ symbols to communicate
across space and time.

Medical Science

Kinesiologic diagnosis is a science in its own right, as reflected by the International College of Applied Kinesiology. Each organ of the body has its corresponding detector muscle, whose weakness signals pathology in the corresponding organ. Kinesiology is already widely used to confirm both diagnosis and the efficacy of a probable therapy. The right dose of the right medicine can also be determined by the patient's kinesiologic response. Similarly, allergies can be detected, and the need for nutritional supplements may be determined.

Research in Theology, Epistemology, and Philosophy

Although the validity of its application may vary with the observer's capacity for awareness, the technique of using kinesiology to ascertain truth itself calibrates at a level of 600 as a methodology. This means that the method described has a degree of reliability that is beyond duality or the realm of ordinary consciousness as we know it in daily life. The level of truth of this book as a whole is approximately 850. To maintain that level throughout, the truth of every chapter, page, paragraph, and sentence has been examined by use of the method described, and all statements and conclusions have been similarly verified.

The confusion surrounding the nature of truth can be mitigated if we calibrate the level of truth of our questions as well as the answers. Paradoxes and ambiguities arise from confusing levels of consciousness; an answer is true only at its own level of consciousness. Thus, we may find that an answer is "correct" but simultaneously "invalid," like a musical note that is correctly played but at the wrong place in the score. All observations are reflections of specific levels of consciousness and are valid only on their own level. Therefore, every means of approaching a subject has its own built-in limitations.

A statement may be true at a high level of understanding, but be incomprehensible to the average mind. Its value may therefore be corrupted when the statement is distorted by the limitations of the listener. This has been the fate of religions throughout the ages, where statements that originated from high levels of awareness are later misinterpreted by followers who are then vested with authority.

Such distortion can be seen to an extreme degree in fundamentalist sects of any religion. The fundamentalist's interpretation of religious teachings, proceeding from negativity, is removed from this negativity only by truth. The lowest depictions of deity are of a god who is jealous, vengeful, and angry, a god of death far removed from the God of mercy and love. The god of righteous negativity represents a glorification of the negative, and provides for followers a disavowal of responsibility through justification of human cruelty and mayhem. In general, pain and suffering increase as one nears the bottom levels of consciousness.

The truth of each level of consciousness is self-verifying in that each level has its native range of perception, which confirms what is already believed to be true. Thus, everyone feels justified in the viewpoints that underlie their actions and beliefs. That is the inherent danger of all so-called "righteousness." Anyone can be righteous, from the killer who justifies his rage, to ecclesiastic demagogues and political extremists of all persuasions. By distorting context, it is possible to rationalize and justify virtually any human behavior.

The human dialogue is awesome in its enormity and subtlety, reflecting the kaleidoscopic interactions of the powerful attractor energy fields that constitute man's consciousness. The brilliance of the world's great philosophers through twenty-five centuries has been staggering in its scope and complexity. Yet, overall there are few areas of agreement as to the nature of truth itself. Without an objective yardstick, every individual who has ever lived has had to sift through the changing reflections of life to discern his own truth; this seems a never-ending struggle to which man is condemned by virtue of his own mental design.

This design predicates that any statement will be true only within a given context, despite the fact that the definitions and derivations of that context are invisible and unstated. It is as though every individual is exploring life with a compass that has a unique setting. That any meaningful dialogue at all is possible bespeaks man's enormous compassion for his own condition and attests that giving cohesion to the whole is an all-inclusive, overarching attractor Field that facilitates the manifestation of the possible into the actual.

Concordance emerges from the organizing patterns hidden behind apparent chaos; thus, the evolution of mankind progresses despite the apparently aberrant signals of individuals at any given moment. Chaos is only a limited perception. Everything is part of a larger whole; everyone is involved in the evolution of the all-inclusive attractor Field of consciousness itself. It is this evolution, innate to the overall Field of consciousness, which guarantees the salvation of mankind, and with it, of all life. The nobility of man is in his constant struggle with his own unasked-for existence in a world that is a house of mirrors—his sole support, his faith in the process of life itself.

CHAPTER 7

Everyday Critical Point Analysis

The potential applications for research we have described thus far give some suggestion about the limitless uses for which this method lends itself. As the interaction of attractor fields of energy with human consciousness reveals itself in the interaction of mind and body, the basic level of available energy in any enterprise can be calibrated. All that is required is two people of integrity, one of whom is familiar with the muscle-testing technique. The practical implications are staggering; this tool can be as germinal to the continuing evolution of society as any of the major discoveries of the physical sciences to date. Let us spell out in more pragmatic detail what this could mean in everyday life.

Inasmuch as the calibrated power of an identified attractor pattern is directly related to its degree of truth, it is possible to cleanly distinguish truth from falsehood, constructive from destructive, the practical and efficient from the unworkable and wasteful. We can identify motive, agenda, and goal in any project or in individuals themselves. Sheep's clothing need no longer hide the wolf.

As we have seen, consciousness reacts decisively to the difference between truth and falsehood. You may instantly reconfirm this by stating your true age, which will make your arm go strong, and then stating your incorrect age, which will make your arm go weak. (Let us say that you are 43 years old.) "I am 43 years old." Having someone press down on your extended arm, you will stay strong. Now say, "I am 45 years old," and you will instantly go weak. Like a computer, consciousness simply answers 0 or 1, true or false. (Any ambiguities in the process are introduced by the questioning method, not the answering mechanism. See Chapter 2, Appendix C, and below.)

We can identify the level of truth of any statement, belief system, or body of knowledge. We may accurately measure the truth of any sentence, paragraph, chapter, or entire book, including this one.[1] We now have available a perspective on social movements and history never before possible. Political research is not confined to the present. We can look back into history to make calibrations, for instance, to compare Gorbachev with Stalin, Trotsky with Lenin, and so on.

In all of these exercises, kinesiology reveals the hidden implicit order by making it explicit, disclosing its true nature. The use of the system is self-educative and self-directing. Each answer, it will be discovered, leads to the next question— happily, in an upward and beneficial direction. We discover the truth about ourselves because our questions themselves are merely the reflections of our own motives, goals, and levels of awareness. It is always informative to calibrate not the answer, but the question.

In discussing the process, we must emphasize again, more specifically, some aspects of the form of questioning. *Precision in wording is of paramount importance.* The question might be posed, for instance, "Is this decision a good one?" But what do we mean by "good"? Good for whom, and in what time frame? Therefore, questions have to be very carefully defined. What we think is good or bad is merely subjective; what the universe "thinks" about it may be quite something else.

Motive in questioning is highly significant. Always ask first, "I may ask this question." Never ask a question unless you are prepared for the answer; the facts may be quite different from what you currently believe. Although there is a potential for emotional upset through the unwise use of this method, experience has shown that continuing the line of inquiry will enlarge the context and heal the disturbance. Let us say a young woman states, "My boyfriend is honest" or "He is good for my life" and the answers are negative. She is disappointed to find that his love is selfish and his interest exploitative. But further questions provide a resolution: "This relationship would end in emotional pain." (Yes.) "I am saving myself a lot of misery now by knowing this." (Yes.) "I can learn from the experience." (Yes.) Thus we see the benefit when the line of inquiry is completed.

On a more mundane level, the same technique can determine whether an investment is an honest one or not, or whether or not an institution can be trusted. We can accurately predict the potential of new developments, not only in marketing, but also in medical research or engineering. We can check the safety precautions being used on great oil tankers. We can judge in advance the advisability of military strategy. We can ascertain who is fit to govern, and distinguish the statesman from the mere politician. In the case of a media event, we can instantly tell whether the interviewer or the interviewee is telling the truth, and, if they are, what level of truth is being expressed. (If you try this during a network news hour, you may have the shocking discovery that, on some occasions, all of the public figures are lying.)

Want to tell if that is a good used car to buy? Easy. If a salesman is telling the truth? Simple. If your new romantic interest is a good bet? Is this a reliable product? Is that employee trustworthy? What is the degree of safety of a new device? Will this device be a success or a flop? What is the integrity, skill, and competence level of a particular doctor or lawyer? Who is the best available therapist, teacher, coach, repairman, mechanic, or dentist? What levels of consciousness are required to properly discharge the duties of specific public offices, and what are the levels of the current incumbents?

This capacity to instantly differentiate truth from falsehood is of such extraordinary potential value to society that we have felt it appropriate in our research to document and verify some explicit practical applications.

Current and Historic Events
Because the technique immediately distinguishes true from false evidence, it can resolve factual disputes— the identity of perpetrators, for instance, or the whereabouts of missing persons. The truth underlying major news events can also be revealed, whether it is the guilt or innocence of contemporary victims and accusers, or the validity of historic conspiracy theories or unsolved mysteries, such as the Amelia Earhart story, the Lindbergh kidnapping, etc. Testimony before Senate hearings and media reports of events are verifiable in a matter of seconds. By use of this technique, for

instance, it will be discovered that a major sports figure who recently served a prison term is actually innocent and his accuser was lying. In another recent prominent case, the accuser is telling the truth and the accused is still holding a high office.

Health Research

The failure to eradicate certain diseases or find their cure is often due to the fact that reason is its own limitation. False answers often preclude searching for true causes. For instance, it is current dogma that tobacco causes cancer; our research, however, revealed that organically grown tobacco tests kinesiologically strong, whereas commercial tobacco tests weak. Tobacco was not noted as a carcinogen before 1957, but it does so now as the result of chemicals introduced into its manufacture at that time. There are other solutions to smokers' lung cancer. Research reported in *Science* in 1995 indicates that one gram per day of vitamin C prevents cell damage from smoking. But the real solution is to identify and remove the carcinogenic chemicals from the manufacturing process.

Criminal Justice and Police Work

To know whether or not a witness is lying is of obvious importance in any case under investigation. But it is equally significant to discover whether the prosecution is withholding evidence or if a jury has been tampered with (or, for that matter, is even capable of understanding the evidence).

One of the most interesting applications of the technique is in crimes where there are no witnesses, and it is the word of the accuser against that of the accused. The rash of allegations of sexual crimes against prominent people is an obvious example. Public figures are easy targets for politically motivated character assassination and, in a society where defendants are treated by the media as if proven guilty merely by virtue of having been accused, they need public protection as much as the accusers.

Statistics and Methodology: Time Saving

Great amounts of money and time are spent gathering data to document what could be discerned in minutes. For instance, to "prove" the validity of the kinesiologic method itself to the skeptical, the following procedures had to be followed: (1) 15 different small groups totaling 360 subjects were tested with both positive and negative stimuli (statistical analysis revealed that $p \leq .001$); (2) 7 large groups totaling 3,293 volunteers were similarly tested ($p \leq .001$); (3) 325 subjects were tested individually ($p \leq .001$); (4) 616 psychiatric patients were tested in groups and individually ($p \leq .001$). The conclusion from all the above was that the null hypothesis was rejected. Traditional methodologies are inefficient.

Politics and Government

Are our leaders telling us the truth? Is a political figure upholding the Constitution of the United States or subverting it for personal gain? Does a particular candidate have the unique capacity to rise to the demands of the office he or she seeks? Are facts being misrepresented by a government agency or spokesperson? Will a proposed policy actually solve the problem for which it has been designed? Such practical issues can now be addressed with certitude. Political debates and public addresses can be analyzed for factuality, and proposed legislation can be assessed from a clearer perspective. Programs that are worthwhile can be definitely identified, and ineffective programs can be dropped.

Commerce

It is possible to diagnose an ailing business or industry and solve its problems without risking financial resources on experiments. Complete analysis of a business starts with calibrating the current and past levels of collective motivation and the abilities of all concerned in its operation. Next, one may calibrate what level needs to be reached by the various departments in order to succeed. Then policies, personnel, products, supplies, advertising, marketing, and hiring procedures can be similarly assessed. Various market strategies can then be investigated without investment in expensive market analysis, which preserves capital while saving enormous amounts of time and energy.

It is wise to remember that in the conventions of commerce, like those of politics, truth has an ambiguous status. There is a universally accepted, implicit understanding that things said to gain advantage are not held to any standard of personal honesty. A convenient conscience regarding the exaggerated claim, the bluff, the white lie, is as much a part of the garb of the marketplace as the business suit and tie. (In fact, intriguingly, kinesiologic analysis commonly tells us no longer to believe an erstwhile trustworthy person once he has donned a suit and tie!) Therefore, numerous applications arise in everyday business—for instance, to determine whether a bill or invoice is accurate. A padded account will make any investigator's arm go weak, as will inferior quality or workmanship. Fraud and bogus imitations are easily detectable; the technique can quickly differentiate a bad check from a good one, a false diamond from a true gem.

Science and Research
The level of truth of any scientific paper, experiment, or theory is easily determinable, a great potential asset to the scientific community and the public at large. The benefits to be derived from a given direction of investigation can be ascertained in advance, as can the value of alternate avenues of research. Examination of the economics of research projects and the capabilities of investigators and equipment is also of practical value.

Critical factor analysis can detect the point in a system at which the least effort is capable of producing the greatest result. Computer simulation, with all its complex and uncertain variables, is the present state-of-the-art technique for predicting developments and exploring alternative proposals. The built-in limitations of logic circuits, however, can be transcended by the kinesiologic use of the world's most advanced computer, the human nervous system. Quantum nonlocality guarantees that the answers to each question are present everywhere, but this fact itself is beyond the comprehension or capability of any conventional computer.

Clinical Work

In medicine, the accuracy of diagnoses, as well as the efficacy of a prescribed treatment, can be tested. The technique is also valuable in psychological issues, where the etiology of a disorder can be quickly ascertained. One currently controversial subject of investigation that obviously suggests itself is the area of so-called repressed childhood memories of alleged sexual abuse. Facts can be quickly differentiated from false "memories" elicited in response to suggestion. Freud concluded that most reports of childhood incest he encountered were of hysterical origin, and he stopped believing them. Then subsequent investigators, however, claimed that the statements of these patients were true. Further research indicated that the reports of the patients' statements as being true were themselves false.

Kinesiologic testing is used to back up clinical judgments, as well as scientifically controlled investigation, because it can transcend the built-in design limitation of double-blind research, which can of itself create the very error it is supposed to prevent. Statistics are no substitute for truth, and in the complexity of bio-behavioral phenomena, proximal antecedents can too easily become classified as ostensible causes. The real "cause" may well be the pull of the future through a hidden attractor field (karma).

Education

A profoundly telling exercise may be performed by evaluating the books in one's library. Simply hold them over your solar plexus, and have somebody test your muscle strength. As you do this, your books will end up in two piles, the true and the false; reflection on the differences between the two can produce a revelation— many testers have found it one of the most valuable experiences of their lives. (Some actually left the two piles there for a long period of time to let the lesson sink in.)

It is equally informative to try the same procedure with one's music collection. The negative group will include violent, sexist rap and heavy metal rock. The positive pile will contain classical music, classic rock (including The Beatles), much country western music, reggae, popular ballads, etc.

Spirituality

Although this chapter has dealt primarily with secular uses of this tool, it should be pointed out that applications of the technique can be profoundly spiritual. We may, for instance, test the contrasting statements: "I am a body," as compared to "I have a body." Appropriate questions proceeding from this point can resolve one's most basic fears. All limiting self-definitions create fear because they create vulnerability. Our perceptions are essentially distorted by our own self-definition, which in turn is qualified by identifying with our limitations. Error occurs when we cling to the belief that I *am* "that." Truth is unveiled when we see that one *has* "that" or *does* "that," instead of *being* "that."

There is great freedom in the realization that I "have" a body and a mind, rather than I "am" my mind or body. Once the fear of death is transcended, life becomes a transformed experience because that particular fear underlies all others. Few people know what it is to live without fear—but beyond fear lies joy, as the meaning and purpose of existence become transparent. Once this realization occurs, life becomes effortless and the sources of suffering dissolve; suffering is only the price we pay for our attachments.

Empirical issues, however, are involved even in spiritual quests. In the matter of spiritual teachers, Americans are extremely naïve, partly because spiritual pursuit does not have a long tradition here as it does in older cultures. That the world abounds with false gurus is well known in India, but such cynicism does not come readily to Americans. Fakes repeatedly come out of India with impressive presentations and hoodwink naïve Western spiritual aspirants who, in childlike trust, leave home and hearth, sell their belongings, and follow the charismatic spiritual con man down a path to eventual disillusionment. The acumen of some of these "gurus" can be dazzling, and their capacity to mimic a convincing sincerity is amazing; they often take in even sophisticated spiritual seekers. This is spiritual seduction. A mixture of truth and falsehood blended in a slick package, the teachings sound valid if one cannot see that their truth has been distorted by a false context.

Such spiritual exploitation is routinely exposed in India, where these media-hungry frauds are held in low regard and often confined to their quarters by the government should they return home. Such so-called "teachers" can inflict terrible suffering and tragedy. The most catastrophic depressions in clinical practice have occurred in people who have discovered that they

have been spiritually deceived and raped. Such disillusionment and pain is far more severe than that which
results from other losses in life, and recovery has not
always been possible.

The charm of all false prophets is persuasiveness.
But use of the testing method described herein provides a foolproof safeguard against such deception. It is
informative to watch TV evangelists with the sound
turned off and have somebody test you. False gurus
also make people go weak in a dramatic fashion. It is as
though the universe considers spiritual rape an especially grave error.

What of a true teacher? In the first place, a universal hallmark is that the true teacher never controls anyone's life in any way—instead, they merely explain
how to advance consciousness. But if we do test, we
will find that Mother Teresa, recognized by the world
through the Nobel Peace Prize, calibrated at 710, and
the acknowledged Indian spiritual saint, Ramana
Maharshi, who died in 1950, calibrated at 720. (He
went into a state of enlightenment at age sixteen, never
left the mountain where he lived, and led a life of humble simplicity, eschewing money, prestige, and followers, and would have remained anonymous had not a
well-known British writer's description of Maharshi's
enlightened state brought seekers from all over the
world.)[2]

Nowhere is spiritual fraud more prevalent than in
the world of channelers and psychics. It is informative
to check out the level of truth these mediums express,
as well as the level of the supposed "source" on the
"other side." Sometimes a surprisingly high level of

truth is in fact being taught. A level of truth that calibrates at 500 is worth listening to—regardless of its
origin—because the inability to love is at the root of
most human problems. Beyond the level of 500, material
possessions and worldly needs become irrelevant,
which is why true teachers neither seek nor desire
material gain.

Appropriate use of the system will always lead to
self-discovery and growth. Eventually, it can lead us to
have compassion for everyone, when we see how we
all must struggle with the downside of human nature.
Everyone is crippled in some area, and everyone is
somewhere on the path of evolution, some ahead of us,
and some behind. In the steps we have walked are the
old lessons of life, and before us are the new teachings
to be learned.

In actuality, there is nothing to feel guilty about and
nothing to blame. There is no one to hate, but there *is*
that which is better avoided, and such blind alleys will
become increasingly apparent. Everyone has chosen
their own level of consciousness, yet nobody could
have done otherwise at any given point in time. We can
only get "there" from "here." Every leap has to have a
platform from which to originate. Pain exists to pro-
mote evolution; its cumulative effect finally forces us in
a new direction, though the mechanism may be very
slow. How many times is it necessary to hit bottom
before a lesson is learned? Perhaps thousands, which
may account for the sheer quantity of human suffering,
so vast as to be incomprehensible. Slowly, by inches,
does civilization advance.

It is an interesting exercise to use the technique to

reassess our society's scapegoats—for example, to calibrate the current power level of the United Nations, and then ask what level would be required to successfully do the job for which it was designed. When we see such discrepancies spelled out in plain numbers, we may stop berating ourselves and blaming institutions, realizing that they often simply do not have the requisite power to accomplish their expected tasks. Condemnation disappears with understanding, as does guilt. All judgment reveals itself to be self-judgment in the end, and when this is understood, a larger comprehension of the nature of life takes its place.

That which is injurious loses its capacity to harm when it is brought into the light. And now nothing need remain hidden. Every thought, action, decision, or feeling creates an eddy in the interlocking, inter-balancing, ever-moving energy fields of life, leaving a permanent record for all of time. This realization can be intimidating when it first dawns on us, but it becomes a springboard for rapid evolution.

In this interconnected universe, every improvement we make in our private world improves the world at large for everyone. We all float on the collective level of consciousness of mankind so that any increment we add comes back to us. We all add to our common buoyancy by our efforts to benefit life. What we do to benefit life automatically benefits all of us because we are all included in that which is life. We *are* life. It is a scientific fact that "what is good for you is good for me."

Simple kindness to one's self and all that lives is the most powerful transformational force of all. It produces no backlash, has no downside, and never leads to loss or despair. It increases one's own true power without exacting any toll. But to reach maximum power, such kindness can permit no exceptions, nor can it be practiced with the expectation of some selfish gain or reward. And its effect is as far-reaching as it is subtle.

In a universe where "like goes to like" and "birds of a feather flock together," we attract to us that which we emanate. Consequences may come in an unsuspected way. For instance, we are kind to the elevator man, and a year later, a helpful stranger gives us a hand on a deserted highway. An observable "this" does not cause an observable "that." Instead, in reality, a shift in motive or behavior acts on a field that then produces an increased likelihood of positive responses. Our inner work is like building up a bank account, but one from which we cannot draw at our own personal will. The disposition of the funds is determined by a subtle energy field, which awaits a trigger to release this power back into our own lives.

Dickens's *A Christmas Carol* is the story of all of our lives. We are all Scrooge. We are all Tiny Tim. All of us are both selfish and lame in some areas. We are all victims like Bob Cratchit, and we are all as indignantly moralistic as Mrs. Cratchit refusing to toast Scrooge. The Ghost of Christmas Past haunts all of our lives; the Spirit of Christmases to Come beckons us all on to make the choices that will enhance both our own existence and that of others. (If we calibrate the energy level of Christmas, by the way, it becomes obvious that its power resides within the human heart itself.)

All avenues of questioning lead to the same ultimate

answer. The discovery that nothing is hidden and truth stands everywhere revealed is the key to enlightenment about the simplest practical affairs and the destiny of mankind. In the process of examining our everyday lives, we can find that all of our fears have been based on falsehood. The displacement of the false by the true is the essence of the healing of all things visible and invisible.

And always a final question will eventually arise for every questioner—the biggest question of all: "Who am I?"

CHAPTER 8

The Source of Power

The ultimate object of our investigation is a practical rather than an academic or philosophic understanding, although certain philosophic conclusions can immediately be drawn from even a brief analysis of power and force. From a practical viewpoint, before proceeding we need to know what the intrinsic source of power is and how it operates. What accounts for its greater strengths? Why is it that force always eventually succumbs to power?

In this respect, the Declaration of Independence can provide a rewarding study. This document calibrates at about 700. If one goes through it sentence by sentence, the source of its power appears: it is the concept that all men are equal by virtue of the divinity of their creation, and human rights are intrinsic to human creation and therefore inalienable. Interestingly enough, this is the same concept that was the source of Mahatma Gandhi's power.

On examination, we will see that power arises from meaning. It has to do with motive, and it has to do with principle. Power is always associated with that which supports the significance of life itself. It appeals to that in human nature which we call noble, in contrast to force, which appeals to that which we call crass. Power appeals to that which uplifts, dignifies, and ennobles. Force must always be justified, whereas power requires no justification. Force is associated with the partial, power with the whole.

If we analyze the nature of force, it becomes readily apparent why it must always succumb to power; this is

153

in accordance with one of the basic laws of physics. Because force automatically creates counter-force, its effect is limited by definition. We could say that force is a movement. It goes from here to there (or tries to) against opposition. Power, on the other hand, stands still. It is like a standing field that does not move. Gravity itself, for instance, does not move against anything. Its power moves all objects within its field, but the gravity field itself does not move.

Force always moves against something, whereas power does not move against anything. Force is intrinsically incomplete and therefore has to constantly be fed energy. Power is total and complete in and of itself and requires nothing from outside of itself. It makes no demands; it has no needs. Because force has an insatiable appetite, it constantly consumes. Power, in contrast, energizes, gives forth, supplies, and supports. Power gives life and energy. Force takes these away. We notice that power is associated with compassion and makes us feel positively about ourselves. Force is associated with judgmentalism and tends to make us feel badly about ourselves.

Force always creates counterforce; its effect is to polarize rather than to unify. Polarization always implies conflict; its cost, therefore, is always high. Because force incites polarization, it inevitably produces a win/lose dichotomy; and because somebody always loses, enemies are always created. Constantly faced with enemies, force requires constant defense. Defensiveness is invariably costly, whether in the marketplace, politics, or international affairs.

In looking for the source of power, we have noted

that it is associated with meaning and that this meaning has to do with the significance of life itself. Force is
concrete, literal, and arguable. It requires proof and
support. The sources of power, however, are beyond
argument and are not subject to proof. The self-evident
is not arguable. That health is more important than
disease, that life is more important than death, that
honor is preferable to dishonor, that faith and trust are
preferable to doubt and cynicism, that the constructive
is preferable to the destructive—are all self-evident
statements not subject to proof. Ultimately, the only
thing we can say about a source of power is that it just
"is."

Every civilization is characterized by native principles. If the principles of a civilization are noble, it succeeds; if they are selfish, it falls. As a term, "principles"
may sound abstract, but the consequences of principle
are quite concrete. If we examine principles, we will
see that they reside in an invisible realm within consciousness itself. Although we can point out examples
of honesty in the world, honesty itself as an organizing
principle central to civilization is nowhere independently existent in the external world. True power, then,
emanates from consciousness itself; what we see is a
visible manifestation of the invisible.

Pride, nobility of purpose, sacrifice for quality of
life—all such things are considered inspirational, giving
life significance. But what actually inspires us in the
physical world are things that symbolize concepts with
powerful meanings for us. Such symbols realign our
motives with abstract principles. A symbol can marshal
great power because of the principle that already

resides within our consciousness.

Meaning is so important that when life loses meaning, suicide commonly ensues. When life loses meaning, we first go into depression; when life becomes less meaningful, then we finally leave it. Force has transient goals; when those goals are reached, there remains the emptiness of meaninglessness. Power, on the other hand, motivates us endlessly. If our lives are dedicated, for instance, to enhancing the welfare of others and everyone we contact, our lives can never lose meaning. If the purpose of our life, on the other hand, is merely financial success, what happens after that has been attained? This is one of the primary etiologies or causes of depression in middle-aged men and women.

The disillusionment of emptiness comes from failing to align one's life with the principles from which power emanates. A good illustration of this phenomenon can be seen in the lives of great musicians, composers, and conductors of our own times. How frequently they continue productive careers into their eighties and nineties, often having children and living vigorously until a ripe old age![1] Their lives have been dedicated to the creation and embodiment of beauty; beauty incorporates and expresses enormous power. We know clinically that alignment with beauty is associated with longevity and vigor. Because beauty is a function of creativity, such longevity is common in all creative occupations.

The philosophic position of reductive materialism, based on the premise that nothing is real unless it is quantifiable, is endemic in the sciences. The source of power, however, is invisible and intangible. The sophistry of logical empiricism is clear from its essential premise. To say that nothing is real unless it is measurable is already an abstract position, is it not? This proposition itself is nowhere tangible, visible, or measurable; the argument of tangibility is itself created from the intangible.

Even if such a position were valid, who would want to live without pride, honor, love, compassion, or value? Despite the pathetic implications of this argument, let us address it nevertheless.

Does power have any tangible basis? Does it proceed exclusively from the undefinable, the mystical, philosophic, spiritual, or abstract? Is there anything more we can know about power that would make sense to those who are oriented only to that left-brain world, which, regardless of its computerized sophistication, remains only a system of mechanical measurements?

Before we proceed, let us remind ourselves that the most advanced artificial intelligence machines in the world are unable to feel joy or happiness. Force can bring satisfaction, but only power brings joy. Victory over others brings us satisfaction, but victory over ourselves brings us joy. But as previous chapters have shown, not only can these qualities now be measured, they can be actually calibrated. To make this fact more comprehensible to reason, let us continue our tour through some easily understood concepts from advanced theoretical physics.

We need not be intimidated by these concepts; on the contrary, their implications for daily life, though profound, are quite simple. We do not have to understand the molecular structure of rubber in order to benefit from having tires on our cars. Although their proofs may be complex, Einstein's Theory of Relativity, Bell's Theorem, and so on, can all be stated in a few easily understandable sentences.

Several recently defined concepts have relevance in understanding the nature of power. One is physicist David Bohm's theory, which states that there is both a visible and an invisible universe.[2] This idea should not be daunting; many things with which we have a daily familiarity—x-rays, radio and TV waves—are not visible either. An "enfolded" universe runs parallel to the visible, "unfolded" universe, which is itself merely a manifestation of that enfolded, invisible universe.

Thus, for instance, did the idea of building the world's tallest building marshal support and result in an invisible concept, which eventually became the Empire State Building within the visible world. The enfolded universe is connected with human consciousness, as inspiration arises in the mind of the creator. Bohm says meaning links mind and matter like opposite sides of a coin.[3]

Another useful concept is Rupert Sheldrake's notion of morphogenetic fields, or M-fields.[4] These invisible organizing patterns act like energy templates to establish forms on various levels of life. It is because of the discreteness of M-fields that identical representations of a species are produced. Something similar to M-fields also exists in the energy fields of consciousness and underlies thought patterns and images—a phenomenon termed "formative causation." The idea that M-fields assist learning has been verified by wide-scale experimentation.[5]

When Roger Bannister broke the four-minute mile, he created a new M-field. The belief system prevailing in human consciousness had been that the four-minute mile was a limit of human possibility. Once the new M-field was created, many runners suddenly began to break the four-minute mile records. This occurs every time mankind breaks into a new paradigm, whether it is the capacity to fly (an M-field created by the Wright Brothers), or the capacity to recover from alcoholism (an M-field created by Bill W., the founder of Alcoholics Anonymous). Once an M-field is created, everyone who repeats the accomplishment reinforces the power of that M-field.

We are all familiar with the fact that new ideas often seem to arise in the minds of several far-removed people at the same time. Somehow, the M-field acts as an organizing principle, like a sort of general magnetic attraction. An M-field does not have to move anywhere. It is a standing energy field that is everywhere present. Once it is created, it exists as a universally available pattern throughout the invisible universe.

The next concept we need to consider in more detail is the so-called chaos theory (nonlinear dynamics). Its first application was in the prediction of weather, the study of which, over the centuries, had established the consensus that there was no definable, predictable mathematical pattern to weather (just as it had also been determined that there was no mathematical way to prove when a dripping faucet will drip, or even to explain how a droplet is formed). Chaos merely means a mass of apparently meaningless data—for instance, a bunch of dots—in which one cannot see any inherent organizing pattern. With the advent of advanced computer technology, it was discovered that inner organizing patterns could be found by computer analysis in what looked like disorganized data; that which appears to be incoherent actually has an inner hidden coherence.

Such analysis revealed patterns that often look like the figure eight folded back upon itself, frequently with a funnel effect, so that the graphic itself has a repeatable geometric configuration. What science has realized is what mystics have claimed throughout the centuries: that the universe is indeed coherent, unified, and organized around unifying patterns.[6]

Nonlinear dynamics has verified that there really is no chaos in the universe; the appearance of disorder is merely a function of the limits of perception. This came as a disturbing revelation to left-brain people, but seemed self-evident to right-brain people. Creative people merely write, paint, sculpt, or design what they already see within their own minds. We do not dance from logic, we dance from feeling patterns. We make our choices from values, and values are associated with intrinsic patterns.

The accepted chain of causality as commonly understood in the basic sciences occurs as the sequence A → B → C. In this scheme of material determinism, nothing is inherently free, but only the result of something else. It is thereby limited; what this system really defines is the world of force. Force A results in Force B, which is then transmitted to Force C with consequence D. D, in turn, becomes the beginning of another series of chain reactions, *ad infinitum*. This is the left-brain world, mundane and predictable. It is the limited paradigm from which the conventional sciences operate: chartable, familiar, controllable, but uncreative—determined, and therefore limited, by the past. It is not the world of genius, but to many it feels safe. It is the world of productivity and practicality. To creative people, however, it seems pedestrian, prosaic, uninspiring, and limiting. It is one thing to conceive of the Empire State Building; it is something else to make it happen. To make a thing happen requires motivation. Motivation is derived from meaning. Therefore, the visible and invisible worlds are linked together, as we have already diagrammed it:

$$ABC$$
$$\downarrow\downarrow\downarrow$$
$$A \rightarrow B \rightarrow C$$

Here we see that the concept ABC, which is within the invisible, enfolded universe, will activate emergence into the visible world to result in the sequence, A → B → C. Thus, the visible world is created from the invisible world, and is therefore influenced by the future.[7] The capacity of the invisible concept to materialize is based on the power of the original concept itself. We might say that the right brain "gets the pattern" and the left brain "makes it visible." An ABC may be either a high-energy attractor or a low-energy attractor. Certain concepts and values apparently have much greater power than others. (Thus far, science has only defined that attractors may have either high energy or low energy.)

Simply stated, powerful attractor patterns make us go strong, and weak patterns make us go weak. Some ideas are so weakening that merely holding them in mind makes test subjects unable to keep their arm up at all. Other concepts are so powerful that when they are held in mind, it is impossible to force down the subject's arm with any amount of exertion. This is a universal clinical observation. Powerful patterns are associated with health; weak patterns are associated with sickness, disease, and even death. If you hold forgiveness in mind, your arm will be very strong. If you hold revenge in mind, your arm will go weak.

For our purposes, it is really only necessary to recognize that power is that which makes you go strong, while force makes you go weak. Love, compassion, and forgiveness, which may be mistakenly seen by some as submissive, are, in fact, profoundly empowering. Revenge, judgmentalism, and condemnation, on the other hand, inevitably make you go weak. Therefore, regardless of moral righteousness, it is a simple clinical fact that in the long run, the weak cannot prevail against the strong. That which is weak falls of its own accord.

Individuals of great power throughout human history have been those who have totally aligned themselves with powerful attractors. Again and again, they have stated that the power they manifested was not of themselves or of their own making. All attributed the source of the power to something greater than themselves.

All of the Great Teachers throughout the history of

our species have merely taught one thing, over and over, in whatever language, at whatever time. All have said, simply: Give up weak attractors for strong attractors.

In examining these attractors, we will notice that some weak patterns tend to imitate (in form only) more powerful patterns. These we will call imitators. Thus, the German people under the Third Reich were deceived by that which appeared to be Patriotism but was really nationalism, that is, patriotism with a small "p." The demagogue or the zealot tries to sell us imitators as the real thing. Demagogues, to this end, put forth a great deal of rhetoric. In contrast, those who move from power need say very little.

PART TWO: WORK

CHAPTER 9

Power Patterns in Human Attitudes

The ability to differentiate between high- and low-energy patterns is a matter of perception and discrimination that most of us learn by painful trial and error. Failure, suffering, and eventual sickness result from the influence of weak patterns; in contrast, success, happiness, and health proceed from powerful attractor patterns. Therefore, it is well worth taking a few minutes to scan the list of contrasting patterns below, which have been researched and calibrated to determine their respective criteria. This listing is an educational tool that operates from the principle of closure. Reflection on the many contrasting pairs of qualities can initiate a consciousness-raising process, so that one gradually becomes aware of patterns operating in relationships, business affairs, and all the various interactions that make up the fabric of life. On the left are adjectives describing powerful (positive) patterns, which calibrate above 200; on the right are weak (negative) patterns, which calibrate below 200.

Abundant	. . .Excessive	Detached	. . .Removed
Accepting	. . .Rejecting	Determined	. .Stubborn
Admitting	. . .Denying	Devoted	. . . .Possessive
Aesthetic	. . . .Artsy	Diplomatic	. .Deceptive
Agreeable	. . . .Condescending	Doing	. . . . . .Getting
Allowing	. . . .Controlling	Educating	. . .Persuading
Appreciative	. .Envious	Egalitarian	. . .Elitist
Approving	. . .Critical	Empathetic	. .Pitying
Attractive	. . . .Seductive	Encouraging	.Promoting
Authoritative	.Dogmatic	Energetic	. . . .Agitated
Aware	. . . . . .Preoccupied	Enlivening	. . .Exhausting
Balanced	. . . .Extreme	Envisioning	. .Picturing
Beautiful	. . . .Glamorous	Equal	. . . . . .Superior
Being	. . . . . .Having	Erotic	. . . . .Lustful
Believing	. . .Insisting	Essential	. . . .Apparent
Brilliant	. . . . .Clever	Eternal	. . . .Temporal
Candid	. . . . .Calculating	Ethical	. . . . .Equivocal
Carefree	. . . .Frivolous	Excellent	. . .Adequate
Challenged	. .Impeded	Experienced	.Cynical
Charitable	. . .Prodigal	Fair	. . . . . . .Scrupulous
Cheerful	. . . .Manic	Fertile	. . . . .Luxuriant
Cherishing	. . .Prizing	Flexible	. . . .Rigid
Choosing-to	. .Having-to	Forgiving	. . . .Condemning
Civil	. . . . . . .Formal	Free	. . . . . . .Regulated
Concerned	.Judgmental	Generous	. . .Petty
Conciliatory	.Inflexible	Gentle	. . . . .Rough
Confident	. . .Arrogant	Gifted	. . . . .Lucky
Confronting	. .Harassing	Giving	. . . . .Taking
Conscious	. . .Unaware	Global	. . . . .Local
Considerate	. .Indulgent	Gracious	. . . .Decorous
Constructive	.Destructive	Grateful	. . . .Indebted
Contending	. .Competing	Harmonious	.Disruptive
Courageous	. .Reckless	Healing	. . . .Irritating
Defending	. . .Attacking	Helpful	. . . . .Meddling
Democratic	. .Dictatorial	Holistic	. . . . .Analytic

Honest . . . . . .Legal		Principled . . .Expedient
Honoring . . . .Enshrining		Privileged . . . .Entitled
Humble . . . . .Diffident		Prolific . . . . . .Barren
Humorous . . .Somber		Purposeful . . .Desirous
Impartial . . . .Righteous		Receiving . . . .Grasping
Ingenious . . . .Scheming		Freeing . . . . . .Tenacious
Inspired . . . .Mundane		Reliant . . . . . .Dependent
Intentional . . .Calculating		Requesting . . .Demanding
Intuitive . . . . .Literal		Respectful . . .Demeaning
Inventive . . . .Prosaic		Responsible . .Guilty
Inviting . . . . . .Urging		Satisfied . . . .Sated
Involved . . . . .Obsessed		Selective . . . . .Exclusive
Joyful . . . . . . .Pleasurable		Serene . . . . .Dull
Just . . . . .Punitive		Serving . . . . .Ambitious
Kind . . . . .Cruel		Sharing . . . . .Hoarding
Leading . . . . . .Coercing		Significant . . .Important
Liberating . . . .Restricting		Sober . . . . . .Intoxicated
Long-term . . . .Immediate		Spontaneous .Impulsive
Loyal . . . . . . .Chauvinistic		Spiritual . . . .Materialistic
Merciful . . . . .Permissive		Steadfast . . . .Faltering
Modest . . . . .Haughty		Striving . . . . . .Struggling
Natural . . . . .Artificial		Surrendering .Worrying
Noble . . . . . . .Pompous		Tender . . . . . .Hard
Nurturing . . . .Draining		Thoughtful . .Pedantic
Observant . . . .Suspicious		Thrifty . . . . . .Cheap
Open . . . . . . .Secretive		Timeless . . . .Faddish
Optimistic . . .Pessimistic		Tolerant . . . .Prejudiced
Orderly . . . . . .Confused		Tractable . . . .Contrary
Outgoing . . . .Reserved		Trusting . . . . .Gullible
Patient . . . . . .Avid		Truthful . . . .False
Patriotic . . . . .Nationalistic		Unifying . . . .Dividing
Peaceful . . . .Belligerent		Unselfish . . .Self-seeking
Polite . . . . . . .Obsequious		Valuing . . . . . .Exploitive
Powerful . . . .Forceful		Virtuous . . . .Celebrated
Praising . . . . .Flattering		Warm . . . . . . .Feverish

Simply reading over this list, you are no longer the same person you were before. Merely to become acquainted with the differences between these polarities begins to increase one's inner power. With these distinctions in mind, we will start to notice things we never observed before. Such revelations occur because, as the reader will discover, the universe favors power.

Moreover, the universe does not forget. There are many sides to the question of karma, but every choice of who and how to be is a choice of great consequence. All of our choices reverberate through the ages. Thousands of reports of near-death experiences have been given over the centuries, as currently reflected in such best-selling books as Dannion Brinkley's *Saved by the Light* or B. J. Eadie's *Embraced by the Light* (which calibrates at 595); these reports confirm that we shall eventually have to accept responsibility for every thought, word, and deed we beget and re-experience exactly whatever suffering we have caused others. It is in this sense that we each create our own heaven or hell.

The universe holds its breath as we choose, instant by instant, which pathway to follow; for the universe, the very essence of life itself, is highly conscious. Every act, thought, and choice adds to a permanent mosaic; our decisions ripple through the universe of consciousness to affect the lives of all. Lest this idea be considered either merely mystical or fanciful, let us remember that fundamental tenet of the new theoretical physics: everything in the universe is connected with everything else.[1]

Our choices reinforce the formation of powerful M-Fields, which are the attractor patterns that influence others.[2] Even if one sits isolated in a cave, his thoughts influence others whether he wishes it or not. Every act or decision you make that supports life supports all of life, including your own. The ripples we create return to us. This, which may once have seemed a metaphysical statement, is now established as a scientific, confirmable fact.[3]

Everything in the universe constantly gives off an energy pattern of a specific frequency that remains for all time and can be read by those who know how. Every word, deed, and intention creates a permanent record. Every thought is known and recorded forever. There are no secrets; nothing is hidden, nor can it be. Our spirits stand naked in time for all to see. Everyone's life, finally, is accountable to the universe.

CHAPTER 10

Power in Politics

To better understand the critical difference between force and power and the implications of this distinction for our own lives, it is helpful to examine human behavior on a larger scale. The interactions of men and governments provide many clear illustrations.

Looking at history from our unique perspective, we will of course be reminded of the powerful example set by the American Revolution, which first formally established freedom as an inalienable right, setting a precedent for centuries to come. Principles that calibrate as high as 700 affect mankind over great courses of time. The pen is indeed mightier than the sword, because power originates from the mind, whereas force is rooted only in the material world.

A related pivotal event in global history, to which we have already referred and will again, came about in this century through the power of a solitary person: Mahatma Gandhi, a ninety-pound so-called "colored" who single-handedly overcame the British Empire, which was then the greatest force in the world, ruling two-thirds of the face of the globe.[1]

Gandhi not only brought the British Empire to its knees, he effectively rang down the curtain on the centuries-old drama of colonialism, and he did it by simply standing for a principle: the intrinsic dignity of man and his right to freedom, sovereignty, and self-determination.[2] Fundamental to this principle, in Gandhi's view, was the fact that such rights derive to man by virtue of the divinity of his creation. Gandhi believed that human rights are not granted by any earthly

173

power, but are inherent in the nature of man himself by consequence of his creation.[3]

Violence is force; because Gandhi was aligned with power instead of force, he forbade all use of violence in his cause.[4] And because he expressed universal principles (which calibrate at 700), he was able to unite the will of the people. When the will of the people is so united and aligned with universal principles, it is virtually unconquerable. Colonialism (which calibrates at 175) is founded on the self-interest of the ruling country. Gandhi demonstrated, for the world to witness, the power of selflessness versus the force of self-interest.[5] (The same principle has also been demonstrated quite dramatically in South Africa by Nelson Mandela.)[6]

Power accomplishes with ease that which force cannot accomplish, even with extreme effort. Thus, in our own time, we have seen the almost effortless toppling of communism as a governmental form, after half a century of the most ominous—and ultimately ineffectual—military confrontation of history. The political naïveté of the Russian people, long used to the tyrannical rule of czars, did not allow them the civic wisdom to understand that in the name of "communism," a totalitarian dictatorship was actually being established. Similarly, the German people were deceived by Hitler, who rose to power in the name of national socialism, only to establish a virtual tyranny. A distinctive characteristic of force in politics is that it cannot tolerate dissent. Both rulers depended on the pervasive use of force through secret police; Joseph Stalin, who also put millions to death, relied on his KGB, as Hitler did his

Gestapo.

Adolf Hitler assembled the greatest military machine the world had ever seen. On the simple level of force, his military was unbeatable; yet he could not defeat a tiny island across the English Channel because of the power expressed by Winston Churchill, who unified the will of his people through principles of freedom and selfless sacrifice. Churchill (calibrated at 510) stood for power, Hitler for force.[7] When power and force meet, power always eventually succeeds; in the long run, if it is deeply founded in the will of the people, power is immune to force.

Force is seductive because it emanates a certain glamour, whether that glamour is manifested in the guise of false patriotism, prestige, or dominance; conversely, true power is often quite unglamorous. What could be more glamorous than the Luftwaffe and the Waffen SS of Nazi Germany during the Second World War? These elite branches embodied romance, privilege, and style, and certainly had enormous force at their disposal—including the most advanced weapons of the day and an *esprit de corps* that cemented their might. Such is the glamour of the formidable.

The weak are attracted to and will even die for the glamour of force. How else could something so outrageous as war even occur? Force often seizes the upper hand temporarily, and the weak are attracted by those who seem to have overcome weakness. How else could dictatorship be possible?

One characteristic of force is arrogance; power is characterized by humility. Force is pompous; it has all the answers. Power is unassuming. Stalin, who strutted military supremacy, has gone down in history as an arch-criminal.[8] In contrast, the humble Mikhail Gorbachev, who wore a plain suit and easily admitted to faults, was awarded the Nobel Peace Prize.

Many political systems and social movements begin with true power, but as time goes on, they become co-opted by self-seekers and end up relying increasingly on force until they finally fall in disgrace. The history of civilization demonstrates this repeatedly. It is easy to forget that the initial appeal of communism was idealistic humanitarianism, as was that of the union movement in the United States, until it became a refuge of petty politicians.[9]

To fully comprehend the dichotomy we are discussing, it is necessary to consider the difference between a politician and a statesman. Politicians, operating out of expediency, rule by force after gaining their position through the force of persuasion and rhetoric—often calibrating at a level less than 200. Statesmen represent true power, rule by inspiration, teach by example, and stand for self-evident principles. Statesmen invoke the nobility that resides within all men and unifies them through what can best be described as "the heart." Although the intellect is easily fooled, the heart recognizes the truth. Where the intellect is limited, the heart is unlimited; where the intellect is intrigued by the temporary, the heart is only concerned with the permanent.

Force often relies upon rhetoric, propaganda, and specious argument to garner support and disguise underlying motivations. One characteristic of truth, though, is that it needs no defense; it is self-evident.

That "all men are created equal" requires no justification or rhetorical persuasion. That it is wrong to gas people to death in concentration camps is self-evident; it requires no argument. The principles upon which true power is based do not require vindication, as force invariably does—there are always endless arguments about whether force is "justified" or not.

It is clear that power is associated with that which supports life, and force is associated with that which exploits life for the gain of an individual or an organization. Force is divisive and, through that divisiveness, weakens, whereas power unifies. Force polarizes. The jingoism that has such obvious internal appeal to a militaristic nation just as obviously alienates the rest of the world.

Power attracts, whereas force repels. Because power unifies, it has no true enemies, although its manifestations may be opposed by opportunists whose ends it does not serve. Power serves others, whereas force is self-serving. True statesmen serve the people;[10] politicians exploit people to serve their own ambitions. Statesmen sacrifice themselves to serve others; politicians sacrifice others to serve themselves. Power appeals to our higher nature, and force to our lower nature. Force is limited, whereas power is unlimited.

Through its insistence that the end justifies the means, force sells out freedom for expediency. Force offers quick, easy solutions. In power, the means and the end are the same, but ends require greater maturity, discipline, and patience to be brought to fruition. Great leaders inspire us to have faith and confidence because of the power of their absolute integrity and alignment with inviolate principles. Such figures understand that you cannot compromise principle and still retain your power. Winston Churchill never needed to use force with the British people; Gorbachev brought about total revolution in the largest political monolith in the world without firing a shot; Gandhi defeated the British Empire without raising a hand in anger. We might note that the seemingly endless Middle-Eastern conflict is not resolvable through violence but eventually, in the long run, through communication.

Democracy and the United States of America

Democracy is eventually being acknowledged universally as the superior form of government. Around the globe, there is a rising call for freedom; many nations with a heritage of repression are learning the lessons necessary for the establishment of liberty. Following conventional science, historians usually try to explain such sequences of political events through an $A \rightarrow B \rightarrow C$ causality; this, however, is merely the apparent sequential unfolding of something with a much greater power, the ABC attractor pattern out of which a society evolves.

The power of the United States, or any other democracy, arises from the principles upon which it is founded. Thus we can find the basis of power by examining such documents as the Constitution of the United States, the Bill of Rights, the Declaration of Independence, and such acknowledged expressions of the spirit of democracy as the Gettysburg Address.

If we calibrate the relative power of each line of

these documents, we find the highest attractor pattern of all, out of which the power of the entire United States government emanates, in the Declaration of Independence: "We hold these truths to be self-evident, that all men are created equal, that they are endowed by their Creator with certain unalienable Rights, that among these are Life, Liberty, and the pursuit of Happiness" (statement calibrates at 700). These sentiments are echoed in the Gettysburg Address, where Abraham Lincoln reminds us that this nation was conceived in Liberty and "...dedicated to the proposition that all men are created equal" and that "this nation, under God, shall have a new birth of freedom—and that government of the people, by the people, for the people, shall not perish from the earth" (also calibrates at 700).

If we examine the actions and statements of Lincoln himself during the years of the Civil War, we will find with certainty that he was devoid of all hatred. He had compassion, rather than malice, for the South, for he understood better than anyone else that the battle was really between man's higher and lower natures. He therefore represented the "self-evident truths" he referred to, and personally mourned the price that he knew had to be paid.[11]

The Declaration of Independence states, "We hold these truths to be self-evident"—that human rights are endowed by nature of man's creation and are inalienable; that is, they do not derive as a fiat from force, nor are they granted by any temporal ruler. Democracy recognizes the divine right of the ruled, rather than the ruler. It is not a right by virtue of title, wealth, or

military superiority, but instead is a profound statement of the essence of man's nature, defining principles
intrinsic to human life itself: liberty and the pursuit of
happiness. (Mahatma Gandhi's power base calibrates
identically with the power base of the Declaration of
Independence and the Constitution; all are essentially
concerned with freedom, liberty, and the equality of all
men by virtue of endowment by a Divine Higher
Power.)[12]

Interestingly, if we calibrate the power of the attractor field of theocracy, we find it consistently lower than
that of any democracy which recognizes the Creator as
the ultimate authority. The makers of the Declaration
of Independence were astute in drawing a very clear
distinction between that which is spiritual and that
which is religious. And they must have intuitively, if
not rationally, known the marked difference between
the power of the two. Religion is often associated with
force, sometimes disastrously so, historically and today;
whereas spiritual concepts such as loyalty, freedom,
and peace do not create strife or conflict, much less
war. Spirituality is always associated with nonviolence.

If we examine the application of the Bill of Rights
today, however, we find that its power in several areas
has dwindled. The right to freedom from unreasonable
search and seizure, as well as freedom from cruel and
unusual punishment, have both been eroded over the
years by expediency. The spirit of the United States
Constitution has become sufficiently dimmed so that
laws which are blatantly unconstitutional are frequently proposed and often passed without a murmur of
protest. Pockets of totalitarianism exist within govern-

ment itself; our society routinely tolerates totalitarian tactics by both federal and local agencies, manifested in the conspicuous use of intimidation. Unfortunately, we have gotten so used to an atmosphere of fear and violence that it comes as a surprise to Americans abroad that the threat of government intrusion or police force does not even exist in many foreign countries.

It is most important to remember that to violate principle for practical expediency is to relinquish enormous power. The rationalization that the execution of criminals deters crime, for instance, does not hold up under study; and the end does not justify the means. The consequence of this violation of principle is reflected in the crime statistics of the United States, where murder is so common it does not even make the front pages.

Because we fail to differentiate principle from expediency, the average person lacks the discernment to understand the difference between patriotism and true Patriotism, between americanism and Americanism, between god and God, between freedom and Freedom, between liberty and Liberty. Thus, "americanism" is used as a justification by white supremacy groups (calibrated at 150) and lynch mobs, just as warmongering throughout history has been conducted in the name of "God." The misinterpretation of liberty as license tells us that many people do not know the difference between freedom as license and true Freedom as principle.

Learning the difference between principles and their imitators requires experience and educated judgment. The exercise of such discretion is necessary for moral survival in the modern world in general, but is imperative in those gray areas, where ethical ambiguity has been elevated from convention to an art form: the political arena and the marketplace of daily commerce.

CHAPTER 11

Power in the Marketplace

Man has freedom of choice, without which there would be no accountability or responsibility. The ultimate choice, really, is whether to align with a high-energy attractor field or a low-energy attractor field. The same weak attractor patterns that have brought down governments, social movements, and entire civilizations routinely destroy organizations and careers. One makes one's choice and then takes the consequences.

Nowhere are these consequences more dramatically visible than in the realm of business. Nowhere else, however, could failure be more easily avoided if a few basic concepts were clearly understood. Attractor fields can be quickly calibrated, whether it is a product, company, advertisement, or employee. In our research, the differences between businesses that have failed and businesses that have succeeded have proved so marked that excellent predictive accuracy can be expected.

All too often, the "buyer"—who can be a voter, investor, or truth-seeker, as well as a purchaser—is captured by the glamour of an imitator pattern that on the surface appears to be a high-energy attractor pattern. People are dazzled by superficial style and slick presentations, like those naïve investors who bought silver only to find that the entire commodity market had been manipulated. Our notorious savings-and-loan fiascoes and their perpetrators could easily have been identified long before the scandals surfaced. Similar disasters can be avoided by simply examining whether a business endeavor is associated with a high or a low attractor pattern. This identification can become almost instinctive once one understands the difference between the operation of force and power in commerce.

Sam Walton, the founder of Walmart, provided a model of how power comes from aligning with high-energy attractor patterns. The ABC that he conceived has resulted in the A→B→C manifestation in the world that is the rapidly growing Walmart colossus. (The basic principles involved are spelled out in the book *Sam Walton* by Vance Trimble.)[1]

In the aisles of many of today's giant stores, there seem to be no employees whatsoever; the gross indifference to customer goodwill is shocking. Walmart's employees, in contrast, are trained to be accommodating, warm, and energetic, to reflect a humane energy field in their workplace. Their jobs have meaning and value because they are aligned with Service, a commitment to the support of life and human value. All Walmart stores feature an area where you can rest your feet and decide about purchases. Such an allocation of space to meet simple human needs would not pass the scrutiny of purely scientific management calculations in terms of gross sales per square footage. But such "efficiency" expertise has discarded, along with human compassion, the market allegiance of millions of customers. Computers do not feel; more attention would be paid to feelings if it were realized that *feelings determine purchases*.

A commercial factor of great, though often unrecognized, importance is the "family" feeling of employees—their loyalty to each other and to their organization. This is a very prominent quality in successful companies. Employees who feel nurtured and supported are those who smile genuinely at customers. Another characteristic of such an environment is low employee turnover, whereas cold and impersonal companies have very rapid employee turnover. Employee shortage is always an expression of a low attractor energy pattern. Critical factor analysis of a large cut-rate drug chain that had just filed for Chapter 11 revealed that the few dollars saved by not having extra employees at the checkout counter regularly cost thousands of dollars in sales; such shortsightedness is common in businesses dominated by low-energy fields.

To be a success, it is necessary to embrace and operate from the basic principles that produce success, not just imitate the actions of successful people. To really do what they do, it is necessary to *be like they are*. Companies that have imitated some of Walmart's features, in hopes of regaining market share, have not been successful because they merely imitated the A→B→C instead of aligning with the ABC that is the core concept from which those features emanated.

Our research on attractor patterns correlates closely with the conclusions arrived at by Thomas Peters and Robert Waterman in their book *In Search of Excellence*, which is a detailed analysis of several great companies.[2] They concluded that successful companies were those that had "heart," as opposed to strictly left-brain, scientifically managed companies. In reading this study, one cannot help but be struck by the inadequacy of many marketing survey procedures; the statisticians simply do not know what questions to ask.

In addition to counting the millions that companies make, analysts might well assess the multimillions that they do not make. A good example is the decline of the U.S. auto industry. One would think that it would be apparent from the success of the Rolls-Royce or the Volkswagen Beetle, that espousing a philosophy of planned obsolescence rather than enduring quality demonstrates a gross miscalculation. Our research indicated years ago that by following the high-energy attractor patterns we have already identified, Detroit could reclaim the auto market. Truly creative innovation is required in order to recapture the imagination of the public, and enduring quality must supplant planned obsolescence, as the price of a new car approaches well over twenty thousand dollars.

Sensibly enough, not many Americans are happy to lay out such sums in full knowledge that the investment will shortly be lost to obsolescence. Obviously, what the depreciating car loses is not any real, innate value: the inflated price of glamour and novelty does not reflect any actual worth. People will gladly pay fifty thousand dollars or more for a used Rolls-Royce, knowing that twenty years from now it will still be classic in style and mechanically sound, with a high re-sale value, maybe even higher than that which they paid in the first place.

Our research indicates that Americans would willingly pay such high prices for cars if their intrinsic worth were equivalent to their purchase price, so as to protect the investment, and, if the cars were to run well and maintain value for a long time, ideally a life-time. (For instance, a modular car in which such items as the motor and drive train were easily removable and replaceable—with a lifetime guarantee—would be a sure winner.) Attractor research tells us that customers are willing to pay for quality, and that good products would sell themselves without slick advertising gim-micks. Integrity and excellence speak for themselves because they are aligned with power.

One of the most profitable and simple applications of critical factor analysis is in the field of advertising. The use of the simple kinesiologic technique we have described can instantly reveal whether an advertising campaign or given commercial makes people go weak or strong.

Companies pay enormous sums to reach the great-est possible audiences, but this strategy can backfire when a widely viewed commercial that makes viewers go weak damages the company's image. An ad that makes people go strong will always produce a positive feeling about the product, rather than an aversion. Similarly, advertisers who buy time during TV programs that make people go weak will find their product unconsciously associated with these negative feelings. By analyzing a commercial in detail, one can ascertain the elements that have a weakening, negative effect— the voice of the announcer; the mannerisms of an actor; or the use of certain words, concepts, or sym-bols. That some companies repeatedly produce taste-less and even embarrassing commercials reflects low attractor fields prevalent in their advertising and marketing departments.

———•———

Beyond the surface world of commerce, society provides numerous other marketplaces where fulfillment
of human needs is sought, bartered, stolen, coerced,
and denied. It is a simple fact of life that satisfaction of
needs brings contentment; frustration breeds violence,
crime, and emotional turmoil. If the mission of government regulatory institutions were realigned to support
the fulfillment of human needs, rather than mounting
moralistic, black-and-white campaigns to stamp out
"social problems," these institutions could become
powerful forces for human betterment.

Perceptual fields are limited by the attractor pattern with which they are associated. This means that
the capacity to recognize significant factors in a given
situation is limited by the context that arises from the
level of consciousness of the observer. The motive of
the viewer automatically determines what is seen;
causality is, therefore, ascribed to factors that are, in
fact, a function of the biases of the observer and are not
at all instrumental in the situation itself. The concept
of "situational ethics" tells us that the right or wrong of
behavior cannot be determined without reference to
context. As each conditioning factor colors the picture,
shades of gray are introduced that alter the significance
of the whole scenario.

One indication of a low-energy attractor field is a
struggle of opposites. Whereas power always results in
a win-win solution, force produces win-lose situations;
the consequent struggle indicates that the correct solution has not been found, as when the assertion of one

group's interests violates those of another, or the rights of the accused conflict with those of the victim. The way to finesse a high-energy attractor field solution is to seek the answer that will make all sides happy and still be practical. Such solutions involve utilization of both the amellorative right brain as well as the judgmental left-brain.

One basic principle has the power to resolve the problems of the social marketplace: support the solution instead of attacking the supposed causes. Attack is in itself inherently a very weak attractor pattern (150), leading through fear to intimidation, coercion and, eventually, moral corruption. The "vice squad" becomes just that, turning city streets into jungles of crime.

Objective examination reveals that most intractable "social problems" appear unsolvable due to the persistence of either sentimentality or juvenile moralizing. Neither of these positions is based on truth, and, therefore, all approaches proceeding from them are weak. Falsehood makes us all go weak; acting from false positions typically results in the use of force. Force is the universal substitute for truth. The gun and the nightstick are evidence of weakness; the need to control others stems from lack of power, just as vanity stems from lack of self-esteem. Punishment is a form of violence, an ineffectual substitute for power. When, as in our society, the punishment rarely fits the crime, it can hardly be effectual; punishment is based on revenge at the weak energy level of 150.

Supporting the solution of human needs, on the other hand, creates a no-cost resolution that brings serenity; attacking the artificially created "problem" is always expensive, in addition to criminalizing society. Only the childish proceed from the assumption that human behavior can be explained in black-and-white terms. Denying basic biologic needs and instinctual drives is futile. Blocking normal sexual outlets merely results in the creation of abnormal sexual outlets. The solutions that have power are the ones realistically based at the level of Acceptance (350) rather than condemnation (150, the level of Anger). In Amsterdam, for instance, one section of the city is traditionally designated as a red-light district, quiet and serene with a pastoral atmosphere; its streets are safe. In Buenos Aires, parts of parks are set aside for lovers. The police patrol these areas in both countries to protect rather than harass, and all is peaceful.

Another example is the previously cited government inability to solve the problem of drug use. Again, the mistake is in looking at the problem moralistically and acting out of force in a punitive role. The original critical error was the failure to differentiate between hard drugs and soft drugs. Hard drugs (narcotics) are addicting, with severe withdrawal effects, and have been traditionally associated with crime. Soft drugs (recreational) are nonaddicting, do not induce withdrawal, and are usually handled initially by amateurs. By criminalizing soft drugs, the government created a new criminal syndicate, wealthy and international in scope. When prohibition was made effective, it created shortages of cheap, relatively harmless drugs on the street which were then quickly replaced by hard-drug merchants, and the peaceful, largely innocuous drug culture became criminalized and vicious.

Successful solutions are based on the powerful principle that resolution occurs not by attacking the negative but by fostering the positive. Recovery from alcoholism cannot be accomplished by fighting intoxication, but, rather, by choosing sobriety. The "war to end all wars" did no such thing, nor could it possibly have done so. Wars, including wars on "vice," "drugs," or any of the basic human needs regularly traded for in the great hidden social marketplace that underlies conventional commerce, can only be won by choosing peace.

CHAPTER 12

Power and Sports

The theoretical understanding at which we have arrived in our study of consciousness provides a context that may be applied to any field of human activity. This can be illustrated by an examination of sports, a good example because sport is so widely observed and extensively documented. Great heroes of sports have been celebrated throughout history at least as much as great figures in science, the arts, or any other area of cultural achievement. Sports figures symbolize for all of us the possibilities of excellence, and, at the level of the champion, mastery.

What is it in athletics that brings a crowd to its feet and commands wildly enthusiastic loyalty? At first, we might think that it is pride, a fascination with competition and triumph. But while these motives may produce pleasure and excitement, they cannot account for the far greater emotions of respect and awe elicited by a display of athletic excellence. What animates the crowd is an intuitive recognition of the heroic striving required to overcome human limitation and achieve new levels of prowess.

High states of consciousness, also, are frequently experienced by athletes. It is well documented that long-distance runners frequently attain sublime states of peace and joy. This elevation of consciousness, in fact, often inspires the prolonged transcendence of pain and exhaustion necessary to achieve high levels of performance. This phenomenon is commonly described in terms of pushing oneself to the point where one suddenly breaks through a performance barrier and the activity then miraculously becomes effortless; the body then seems to move with grace and ease of its own accord, as though animated by some invisible force. The accompanying state of joy is quite distinct from the thrill of success; it is a joy of inner peace and oneness with all of life.

It is notable that this transcendence of the personal self and surrender to the very essence or spirit of life often occur at a point just beyond the apparent limit of the athlete's ability. The seeming barrier is predicated by the paradigm of one's own past accomplishments or of what has been recognized as theoretically possible, such as the historic "four-minute mile." Until Roger Bannister broke the four-minute mile, it was universally accepted that it was not humanly possible to run any faster than that; Bannister's greatness was not just in breaking the record, but in breaking through that paradigm to a new model of human possibility. This breakthrough to new levels of potential has correspondences in every field of human endeavor; in many diverse enterprises, those who have achieved greatness have given parallel accounts of the circumstances surrounding their accomplishments.

We have made calibrations of various kinds of records of athletic achievement and other areas of human endeavor such as movies. Of all the movies about sport studied, the French film *The Big Blue* produced the highest calibration.[1] This is the story of the world's deep-sea diving champion, Jacques Mayol, the Frenchman who until recently held the world record. The movie calibrates at the extraordinary energy level of 700 (that is, the oneness of all of life, and universal truth), and has the capacity to put viewers into a high state of consciousness; the manager of one movie theater that showed it described audiences wandering out of the theater lost in silence or crying with an inner joy that she had never seen before and could not describe.

The movie achieves an accurate depiction of the world's greatest deep-sea diver in elevated states of consciousness through the use of slow-motion photography. A subjective sensation of slow motion, beauty, and grace is frequently noted in higher states; time seems to stop, and there is an inner silence, despite the noise of the world.

We see throughout the film that Jacques Mayol maintains this state by the intensity of his concentration, which keeps him in an almost constant meditative condition. In this mode, he transcends ordinary human limitations, enabled to achieve great feats through altered physiology. The deeper he dives, the slower his heartbeat becomes, and his blood distribution concentrates almost entirely in his brain (as does that of the porpoise). His best friend in the movie, himself a highly evolved athlete, dies in the attempt to match Mayol's feat because he had not reached the level of consciousness required to transcend the normal limits or requirements of the body.

The subjective experience of effortless bliss also occurs in other types of exceptional physical performance, such as that of the world-famous Sufi dancers known as whirling dervishes, who, through discipline and exhausting practice, become able to move effortlessly through space over long periods of time with dazzling precision.

The most highly developed martial arts clearly demonstrate how motive and principle are of ultimate importance in extraordinary athletic achievement.[2] The most frequently heard admonition to trainees is: "Stop trying to use force."[3] Schools devoted to these arts produce masters whose overriding concern is victory of the higher self over the lower self through control, training, and commitment to goals aligned with true power.[4] Alignment with these high-power attractor patterns is not limited to the exercise of the discipline itself but becomes an entire lifestyle. Thus, when the power of the principle is transferred to the practitioners, the results begin to be manifested everywhere in their life.

The hallmark of true greatness in athletic achievement is always humility (such as that exhibited by Pablo Morales after winning his Gold Medals in the 1992 Summer Olympics). Such athletes express gratitude, inner awe, and an awareness that their performance was not merely the result of personal effort—that maximum personal effort brought them to the breakthrough point from which they were then transported by a power greater than that of the individual self. This typically is expressed as the discovery of some aspect of the greater Self hitherto unknown, or unexperienced in its pure form.

Through kinesiology, we can demonstrate that if one is motivated by any of the energy fields below Courage, one goes weak. The notorious Achilles' heel that brings down not just athletes but also the potentially great in all areas of human achievement is Pride. Pride, calibrated at 175, not only makes the performer go weak, but it cannot provide the motivational power of love, honor, or dedication to a higher principle (or even to excellence itself). If we ask a powerful athlete to hold in mind the hope of defeating his opponent, or becoming a star, or making a lot of money, or becoming famous, we will see that he goes weak and we can put down his trained, muscular arm with minimal effort. The same athlete holding in mind the honor of his country or his sport, the dedication of his performance to someone he loves, or even the sheer joy of maximum effort for the sake of excellence, goes powerfully strong, and we cannot push down his arm with even the greatest effort.

Thus, the competitor who is motivated by pride or greed, or interested primarily in defeating an opponent, will go weak at the moment of the starting gun and be unable to achieve the maximum continued effort necessary for great achievement. At times, we see an athlete start badly for such reasons, but, as the contest progresses and selfish goals are forgotten, we see an improvement in his performance. We also see the opposite happen when an athlete starts well because he is competing for the honor of his country, his team, or of the sport itself, but then falters as he nears the goal, as the anticipation of personal glory or triumph over a rival makes him lose strength and form.

One unfortunate sequence of consciousness occurs when an athlete sets a new record during qualifying trials, arousing new personal ambitions, and then during the final competition, goes to pieces to the puzzlement of the audience. If top performers are imbued with the knowledge that their excellence is not a personal accomplishment, but a gift belonging to all of mankind as a demonstration of man's potential, they will go strong and remain so throughout the whole event.

The scale of consciousness may be seen in one aspect as a scale of ego, with the level of 200 being the fulcrum at which selfishness begins to turn to selflessness. At the rarefied plane of Olympic competition, the disastrous consequences, both in private and in public life, of motivations emanating from levels below 200 are all too clearly illustrated by the scandals at the time. Excessive zeal to capture an Olympic medal and defeat one's opponent by any means available has led to the abandonment of the power of ethical principle and a descent to the grossest level of force. There could hardly be a more telling example of how submission to a negative attractor field can produce a rapid collapse of an otherwise promising athletic career.

Where higher motivations toward excellence give access to the realm of grace and power, self-centered motivations of personal gain draw one almost magnetically into the realm of force. The reaping of recognition—even in the symbolic form of a medal, let alone the financial reward that may accompany it—has little to do with true athletic greatness, which proceeds from an attainment of stature of the spirit; it is this that we laud in the champion. Even if the competitor does not surrender to the lust for wealth and fame, the drive to attain dominance in one's sport, rather than to simply manifest all the excellence of which one is capable, has its own corrupting, egocentric effect—entrainment by the negative forces associated with the level of Pride.

There is nothing intrinsically wrong with some manifestations of pride. We all may well be proud when we take the America's Cup or our Olympians win medals, but that is a different kind of pride. It is an honoring of human achievement that transcends personal pride. We honor the endeavor, not the personal accomplishment, which is only the occasion and expression of something greater, universal and innate in the human heart. The Olympics, one of the greatest dramas of human striving, and one that captures everyone's imagination, provide a context that should counteract personal pride. The whole setting inspires the competitor to move from personal pride to an esteem that is an expression of unconditional love and that honors one's opponents, as well, for their dedication to the same lofty principles.

The media tend to evoke the downside of sports and undermine the athlete, because celebrity status either consciously or unconsciously elicits this egotism. Great athletes need to gird themselves against this source of contamination. Humility and gratitude seem to be the only effective shields against the onslaughts of media exploitation. Athletes in the traditional martial arts employ specific exercises to overcome any tendency toward egotism. The dedication of one's skill, performance, or career to a higher principle provides the only absolute protection.

True athletic power is characterized by grace, sensitivity, inner quiet, and paradoxically, gentleness in the noncompetitive lives of even fierce competitors. We celebrate the champion because we recognize that he has overcome personal ambition through sacrifice and dedication to a higher principle. The great become legendary when they teach by example. It is not what they have, nor what they do, but what they have become that inspires all of mankind, and it is that which we honor in them. We should seek to protect their humility from the forces of exploitation that accompany acclaim in the everyday world. We need to educate the public that the abilities of these athletes and their great performances are gifts to mankind to be respected and defended from the abuse of the media and corporate commerce.

The Olympic spirit resides within the heart of every man and woman. Great athletes can, by example, awaken awareness of those principles in all people. These heroes and their spokesmen have a potentially powerful influence on all of mankind, literally the power to lift the world on their shoulders. The nurturing of excellence and recognition of its value is the responsibility of all men, because the quest for excellence in every area of human endeavor inspires us all toward the actualization of every form of man's yet unrealized greatness.

CHAPTER 13

Social Power and the Human Spirit

When we cheer the spirit of the true athlete, what we applaud is a demonstration of all the significances the word "spirit" entails for us: courage, tenacity, commitment, alignment with principle, demonstration of excellence, honor, respect, and humility.[1] To inspire implies filling with spirit; dispirited means dejected, hopeless, defeated. But what exactly does the term "spirit" signify? The collective totality of human experience can be comprehended by *spirit* in phrases such as "team spirit" or when we exhort people to "get in the spirit." That spirit is a highly pragmatic factor, which can determine the difference between victory and defeat, is well known by military commanders, coaches, and CEOs. Employees or other group members who do not enter into the spirit of the group enterprise soon find themselves without a job or group.

From all of the above it is clear that the term "spirit" refers to an unseen essence and that, although its expression varies from one situation to another, the essence itself never changes.[2] This essence is vital; when we lose our spirit, we die—we expire from lack of that which inspires.

Clinically speaking, then, we can say that spirit equates with life; the energy of life itself can be termed spirit. Spirit is the aliveness that accompanies and is the expression of alignment with life energy. The power of high-energy attractor patterns is anabolic, sustaining life; their opposites are catabolic, eventually leading to death. True power equals life equals spirit, whereas force equals weakness equals death. When an individual has lost or lacks those qualities we term spiritual, he becomes devoid of humanity, love, and self-respect; he may even become selfish and violent. When a nation veers from its alignment with the spirit of man, it can become an international criminal.

It is a common error to identify spirituality with religion. We have noted that the United States Constitution, the Bill of Rights, and the Declaration of Independence clearly differentiate between the spiritual and the religious. The United States government is forbidden to establish any religion, lest it impair the freedom of the people; yet these same documents presume that government's authority derives essentially from spiritual principles.[3]

In fact, the founders of the world's great religions would be shocked at the profoundly unspiritual deeds wrought in their names throughout history—much that would make a heathen shudder. Force always distorts truth for its own self-serving purpose. Over time, the spiritual principles upon which religions are based become distorted for expedient ends, such as power, money, and otherworldliness. Whereas that which is spiritual is tolerant, religiosity is commonly intolerant; the former leads to peace—the latter to strife, bloodshed, and pious criminality. There remains, however, buried within every religion, the spiritual foundation from which it originated.[4] Like religions, entire cultures are weakened when the principles on which they are based are obscured or contaminated by false interpretation.

To more fully understand the nature of spirit in

power and how it originates and operates as a social movement, we will do well to study a contemporary spiritual organization of enormous power and influence, about which everything is of public record, and one that is avowedly aligned with the spirit of man, yet flatly states that it is not religious. This example is the 55 year-old organization known as Alcoholics Anonymous (AA).

In our society we have all gotten to know something about Alcoholics Anonymous, because it has become woven into the very fabric of modern society and its adherents number in the millions. AA and its offshoot organizations have been estimated to affect, in one way or another, the lives of about 50 percent of Americans at this time. Even where the 12-step-based self-help groups do not enter lives directly, they affect everyone indirectly because they reinforce certain values by example. Let us study the power principles upon which AA is based and how this foundation came about historically, and examine the impact that these principles have within the general population, as well as among members. We can look at what AA is and also what it is not, and learn from both.

According to its preamble, AA is "not allied with any sect, denomination, politics, or organization." It has "no opinion on outside matters." It is neither for nor against any other approach to the problem of alcoholism. It has no dues or fees, no ceremonies, trappings, officers, or laws. It owns no property; it has no edifices. Not only are all members equal, but all AA groups are autonomous and self-supporting.[5] Even the 12 basic steps by which members recover are described as only "suggestions." The use of coercion of any kind is avoided, and this is emphasized by slogans such as "Easy does it," "First things first," and, most important, "Live and let live."[6]

Alcoholics Anonymous respects freedom, in that it leaves choice up to the individual. Its identifiable power patterns are those of honesty, responsibility, humility, service, and the practice of tolerance, good-will, and brotherhood. AA does not subscribe to any particular ethic, has no code of right and wrong or good and bad, and avoids moral judgments. AA does not try to control anyone, including its own members. What it does instead is chart a path. It merely says to its members, "If you practice these principles in all of your affairs, you will recover from this grave, progressive, incurable, and fatal illness, and you will regain your health and self-respect, and the capacity to live a fruit-ful and fulfilling life for yourself and others."[7]

AA is the original example of the power of these principles to cure hopeless disease and change the destructive personality patterns of members. From this original paradigm came all subsequent forms of group therapy, through the discovery that groups of people coming together on a formal basis to address their mutual problems have enormous power: Al-Anon for the spouses of AA members; then Alateen for their children; then Gamblers Anonymous, Narcotics Anonymous, Parents Anonymous, Overeaters Anonymous, and so on. There are now close to 300 anonymous 12-step self-help organizations dealing with every aspect and form of human suffering. Americans, as a result of all of this, have now largely turned from condemning self-destructive behaviors to recognizing that these conditions are indeed curable illnesses.

From a practical viewpoint, the sizable impact of self-help organizations on society can be counted, not only in the relief of human suffering and the reconstitution of families, but also in the savings of billions of dollars. Absenteeism, automobile insurance rates, welfare, health care, and penal system costs are all greatly moderated by the widespread behavioral change produced by this movement. The cost of state-provided counseling and group therapy alone for the millions of troubled individuals served would be staggering.

The members of these organizations, collectively by the millions, unanimously agree that admitting the limitations of their individual egos allowed them to experience a true power, and that it is that power which brought about their recovery—which hitherto nothing on Earth, including medicine, psychiatry, or any branch of modern science, had been able to effect.

We can make some important observations from the story of how the prototype 12-step organization, Alcoholics Anonymous, came into existence. Back in the 1930s, alcoholism was accepted, as it had been over the centuries, as a hopeless, progressive disease that had baffled medical science, and religion as well. (In fact, the prevalence of alcoholism among the clergy itself was alarmingly high.) All forms of drug addiction were thought to be incurable, and when they reached a certain stage, victims were simply "put away."

In the early 1930s, a prominent American business-

man (known to us as Rowland H.) who had sought
every cure for his alcoholism without avail, went to see
the famous Swiss psychoanalyst Carl Jung. Jung treated
Rowland H. for approximately a year, by which time he
had achieved some degree of sobriety. Rowland
returned to the United States full of hope, only to fall ill
again with active alcoholism.

Rowland went back to Switzerland to see Jung
again and ask for further treatment. Jung humbly told
him that neither his science nor his art could help him
further, but that throughout man's history—rarely, but
from time to time—some people who had abandoned
themselves completely to some spiritual organization
and surrendered to God for help had recovered.[8]

Rowland returned to the United States dejected,
but he followed Jung's advice and sought out an organization of that time called the Oxford Groups. These
were groups of individuals who met regularly to discuss living life according to basic spiritual principles,
very much like those adopted later by AA. Through
these means, Rowland in fact recovered, and his
recovery was a source of astonishment to another
concerned party named Edwin T., or "Ebby," who was
also an alcoholic, hopeless beyond all help. When
Rowland told Ebby of how he had recovered, Ebby
followed suit and also got sober. The pattern of one
person helping another with the same problem then
extended from Ebby to his friend Bill W., who had
been hospitalized frequently for hopeless, incurable
alcoholism and whose condition was medically grave.
He was described as hopeless. Ebby told Bill that his
recovery was based on service to others, moral house-

cleaning, anonymity, humility, and surrendering to a power greater than oneself.[9]

Bill W. was an atheist, and found the idea of surrendering to a higher power unappealing, to say the least. The whole idea of surrender was abhorrent to Bill's pride; he sank into an absolute, black despair. He had a mental obsession with, and a physical allergy to, alcohol—which condemned him to sickness, insanity, and death, a prognosis that had been clearly spelled out to him and his wife, Lois. Ultimately, Bill gave up completely; at this point he had the profound experience of an infinite Presence and Light and felt a great sense of peace. That night, he was finally able to sleep, and when he awoke the next day, he felt as though he had been transformed in some powerful, indescribable way.[10]

The validity and efficacy of Bill's experience was confirmed by Dr. William D. Silkworth, his physician on the west side of New York City. Silkworth had treated ten thousand alcoholics and, in the process, had acquired enough wisdom to recognize the profound importance of Bill's experience. It was he who later introduced Bill to the great psychologist William James's classic book, *The Varieties of Religious Experience*.

Bill wanted to pass his gift on to others, and as he himself said, "I spent the next few months trying to sober up drunks, but without success." Eventually, he discovered that it was necessary to convince the subject of the hopelessness of his condition—in modern psychological terms, to overcome his denial. Bill's first success was Dr. Bob, a surgeon from Akron, Ohio, who turned out to have a great aptitude for the spiritual and became a co-founder of AA. He never took another drink until his death in 1956 (neither did Bill W., who died in 1971.)[11] The enormous power that was realized through Bill W.'s inner experience has manifested itself externally in the millions of lives that have been transformed because of it. In *Life Magazine*'s listing of the 100 greatest Americans who ever lived, Bill W. is credited with being the originator of the entire self-help movement.[12]

The story of Bill W. is typical of individuals who have been channels of great power: the principles they convey in a brief career reorder the lives of millions over long periods of time. Jesus Christ, for instance, taught for only three short years, and yet his teachings transformed all of Western society for the generations since; man's encounter with these teachings lies at the center of Western history for the last two thousand years. The highest calibrations of attractor power fields that we have discovered have invariably been associated with the teachings of the greatest spiritual masters of history.

There is always a diminution from the calibrated power of the energy field of the original teachings of the great masters to their current practice in the form of organized religion (see Chapter 23). Yet the original principles themselves retain their innate attractor power pattern; it is merely their expression that has become weaker. The teachings themselves have the same profound power they always did.

The power of a principle remains unchanged throughout time. Whether we fully understand them or not, these principles are the ideals for which mankind strives. From our own struggles to better ourselves, we learn compassion for those still in the grip of inner conflict; out of this grows a wisdom, including compassion, for the entire human condition.

If we refer to the principles of advanced theoretical physics, and the results of our own attractor research, it will be obvious that in a universe in which everything is connected with everything else, unseen power accomplishes for us things that we could never do by ourselves. As we have said before, we cannot see electricity, x-rays, or radio waves, but we know of their intrinsic power by virtue of their effects. Similarly, we constantly observe the effects of power in the world of thoughts and feelings, although until now, it has not been considered possible to measure the energy or power of a thought.

When we discuss high-power attractor fields, we frequently can allude to them only by means of symbols. National flags are just dyed patterns on pieces of material, from a physical viewpoint, but men are willing to die for what they symbolize. Empowerment, as we have said, comes from meaning. Those things that have the greatest meaning to us arise from the spiritual, not the material, world.

Thus far, we have seen that alignment with the principles associated with high-power attractor energy fields can result in Olympic achievement; success in commerce; political victory on an international level; and recovery from hopeless, progressive diseases. These same attractor patterns are responsible for the finest music ever written. They are the basis of the most eminent religious teachings, the world's greatest art and architecture, and the wellspring of all creativity and genius.

CHAPTER 14

Power in the Arts

The great works of art, music, and architecture that have come down to us through the centuries are enduring representations of the effect of high-energy attractor patterns. In them, we see a reflection of the commitment of the master artists of our civilization to perfection and grace, and thereby to the ennoblement of humanity.

The fine arts have always provided the venue for man's highest spiritual strivings in the secular realm. As far back as the time of the sculptor Phidias in ancient Greece, it has been the role of the arts to realize, in physical media, the ideals of what man could and should be, to set down in tangible form, accessible to all, a distilled expression of the human spirit.

Great art bodies forth the ordered essence not only of human experience, but of the world we live in. It is this that we call beauty. Like the theoretical physicist, the artist finds order in apparent chaos. Where there was only a block of meaningless marble, Michelangelo saw *David* and the *Pietà*, and with his chisel, removed the extraneous stone to liberate that perfected image. Contemplating the random patterns of a meaningless plaster wall in the Sistine Chapel, he conceived through the inspiration of Art a wondrous ABC, and then through the technique of art, he actualized A→B→C, which we know as *The Last Judgment*.

The bequest of the arts to mankind is internal, too: in beholding realized beauty, a sensitivity to the beautiful is inculcated in us, enabling us to discover, and create, our own aesthetic rewards in the apparently disordered jumble of existence. Art and Love are man's greatest gifts to himself.

There is no art without love. Art is always the making of the soul, the craft of man's touch, whether that touch is corporeal or the touch of the mind and spirit; so it has been since Neanderthal times, and so it will always be. Thus, we find that computer-generated art and even great photographs never calibrate as highly as original paintings. A most interesting kinesiologic experiment, which anyone can reduplicate, is to test the strength of a person who is looking at an original painting and then repeat the test looking at a mechanical reproduction of that painting. When a person looks at something that has been handcrafted, he goes strong; when he looks at a reproduction, he goes weak, and this is true regardless of pictorial content. An original of a disturbing subject will make the test-subject go stronger than a copy of a pleasant subject. Dedicated artists put love into their work, and there is great power in both the human touch and human originality. Therefore, kinesiology provides a fail-safe detector of art forgery.

The great psychoanalyst Carl Jung emphasized over and over again the relationship of art to the dignity of man and the importance of the human spirit in art. Jung himself (and his work) calibrate highest out of all the famous psychoanalysts in history. (Many of the others, aligned with such attractor patterns as material determinism, produced much lower scores.)

Music is in some ways the most subtle, in that it is the least concrete of the arts. However, in bypassing left-brain rationality to appeal directly to our subcon-

scious right-brain sense of pattern, it is at the same time
the most visceral and emotional. It also provides the
easiest example of how attractor patterns order reality:
if you wish to comprehend the difference between
chaos and meaning, thereby attaining an effective definition of art, simply contemplate the difference
between noise and music.

A description of the creative process by the contemporary Estonian composer Arvo Pärt, whose work
is often described as "transcendental" or "mystical,"
condenses much of what we have observed regarding
the crucial role of artistic genius in the unfoldment of
attractor patterns:

> To write, I must prepare myself for a long
> time. Sometimes it takes five years.... In my
> life, my music, my work, in my dark hours, I
> have the certain feeling that everything out-
> side this one thing has no meaning. The
> complex and many-faceted only confuses
> me, and I must search for unity. What is it,
> this one thing, and how do I find my way to
> it? Traces of this thing appear in many guises
> and everything that is unimportant falls
> away.... Here I am alone with silence. I have
> discovered that it is enough when a single
> note is beautifully played....That is my goal.
> Time and timelessness are connected. This
> instant and eternity are struggling within
> us.[1]

Among the arts, it is music that most readily brings
tears to our eyes, or brings us to our feet, or inspires us
to pinnacles of love and creativity. We have already

noted that longevity seems to be a corollary of association with the attractor fields of classical music, whether as performer, conductor, or composer. Classical music often demonstrates extremely high inherent power patterns.

Of all the arts, architecture is the most tangible and influential in the lives of men everywhere. We live, shop, go to work, and seek our entertainment in buildings; thus, the form of the structure itself, because its influence is a background to so much human activity, deserves the utmost attention.

Of all the world's architecture, the great cathedrals elicit a special awe. Their energy patterns have calibrated the highest among architectural forms. This appears to be the result of several factors. Our experience of cathedrals can combine a number of arts simultaneously: music, sculpture, and painting, as well as spatial design. Moreover, these edifices are dedicated to the Divine; that which is begotten in the name of the Creator is aligned with the highest attractor patterns of all. The cathedral not only inspires, but unifies, teaches, symbolizes, and serves all that is noblest in man.

Beauty in architecture, however, need not be expansive or grand in scale. There are few architectural settings more charming than the little thatched cottages dotting the Irish countryside, each one more quaint and picturesque than the last. Innate appreciation for the aesthetic allows in much traditional domestic architecture elegant statements of beauty via simplicity.

Well-conceived public architecture speaks with historical authenticity of the beauty of line combined with utility. Function and beauty are impressively joined in the great subway stations of Russia and in the design and layout of many new high-rise apartment buildings in Canada. Older cultures seem always to have known the practicality of beauty: that which is designed without beauty quickly deteriorates. An architecturally ugly neighborhood becomes part of a feedback loop of blight and violence; the sleazy, dehumanized housing projects of urban ghettos manifest their weak power patterns as a matrix of squalor and crime—although it must be remembered that depending on which attractor pattern one aligns with, the destitution of the ghetto can be an excuse for depravity or the inspiration to rise above it. (It is not the facts of one's environment, but one's attitude toward them, that determines whether they will be the occasion for defeat or the inspiration to victory.)

Grace is the expression of the power of aesthetic sensitivity, and power is always manifested with grace, whether in beauty of line or style of expression. We associate grace with elegance, refinement, and economy of effort. We marvel at the grace of the Olympic athlete, just as we are uplifted by the grace of the Gothic cathedral. Gracious power patterns acknowledge and support life. They respect and uphold the dignity of others. Grace is an aspect of unconditional love. Graciousness also implies generosity—not merely material generosity, but generosity of spirit, such as the willingness to express thanks or acknowledge the importance of others in our lives. Grace is associated with modesty and humility. Power does not need to flaunt itself, though force always must because it originates in self-doubt. Great artists are thankful for their power, whatever its expression, because they know it is a gift for the good of mankind, entailing responsibility to others.

Beauty has expressed itself in so many different forms in different cultures throughout various periods of time that we have good reason to say it is in the eye of the beholder. However, we should note that it is only the vehicle of beauty that changes; the essence of beauty does not change, only the form in which it is perceived. It is interesting that people of advanced consciousness are able to see beauty in all forms. To them, not only is all life sacred, but all form is beauty.

CHAPTER 15

Genius and the Power of Creativity

Creativity and genius are the center of powerful, high-energy attractors. No human talents are more germane to the creation of new M-fields or the unfoldment of the enfolded universe; in fact, these are the explicit domain of creativity and genius. Yet these closely allied processes remain shrouded in mystery; there is a paucity of information about the essential nature of either creativity or genius.

Human history is the record of man's struggle to comprehend truths which to those of genius appear obvious. Genius is by definition a style of consciousness characterized by the ability to access high-energy attractor patterns. It is not a personality characteristic. It is not something that a person "has," or even something that someone "is." Those in whom we recognize genius commonly disclaim it. A universal characteristic of genius is humility. The genius has always attributed his insights to some higher influence.

The process of animating genius most commonly involves first formulating a question, and waiting an indefinite interval for consciousness to work with the problem; then, suddenly, the answer appears in a flash, in a form that is characteristically nonverbal. Great musicians throughout history have stated that they did not plan their music, but rather wrote down what they heard, finished, within their own minds.[1] The father of organic chemistry, F.A. Kekulé, saw the pattern of the carbon ring organic nucleus in a dream. In an illuminated moment, Albert Einstein had the revolutionary insight that then took him years to translate into provable mathematics.[2] Indeed, one of the main problems of genius is how to transform that which is perceived in one's private understanding into a visible expression that is comprehensible to others. The revelation itself is usually complete and self-explanatory to the person who receives it, but to make it so to others may take a lifetime.[3]

Genius, thus, seems to proceed from sudden revelation rather than from conceptualization, but there is an unseen process involved. Although the genius's mind may appear stalled and frustrated with the problem, what it is really doing is preparing the field. There is a struggle with reason that eventually leads, like a Zen koan, to a rational impasse from which the only way forward is by a leap from a lower to a higher attractor energy pattern.

Attractor energy patterns have harmonics, as do musical tones. The higher frequency the harmonic, the higher the power. What the genius arrives at is a new harmonic. Every advance in human consciousness has come through a leap from a lower attractor pattern to a higher harmonic. Posing the original question activates an attractor; the answer lies within its harmonic. This is why it is said that the question and the answer are merely two sides of one coin, and that one cannot pose a question unless the answer already exists—otherwise, there would be no pattern from which the question could be formulated.[4]

Recognized geniuses may be rare, but Genius resides within all of us. There is no such thing as "luck" or "accident" in this universe. And not only is everything connected to everything else, but no one is excluded from the universe. We are all members. Consciousness is a universal quality, like the quality of physicality. Because genius is a characteristic of consciousness, genius is also universal. That which is universal is, therefore, theoretically available to every man.

The processes of creativity and genius are inherent in human consciousness. Inasmuch as every human has within himself the same essence of consciousness, genius is a potential that resides within everyone. It awaits only the right circumstances to express itself. Each of us has had moments of genius in our lifetimes, perhaps only known to ourselves or to those closest to us. We suddenly make a brilliant move or decision, or say exactly the right thing at the right moment, without really knowing why. Sometimes we would like to congratulate ourselves for these fortuitous events, but in truth we really do not know from whence they come.

Genius is often expressed through a change of perception—a change of context or paradigm. The mind struggles with an insoluble problem, poses a question, and is open to receive an answer. The source from which this answer comes has been given many names, varying from culture to culture and from time to time; in the arts of Western civilization, it has traditionally been identified with the Greek goddesses of inspiration called the Muses. Those who are humble and grateful for illumination received continue to have the capacity to access genius. Those who arrogate the inspiration to their own ego soon lose this capacity, or are destroyed by their success. High power, like high voltage, must be handled with respect.

Genius and creativity, then, are subjectively experienced as a witnessing. It is a phenomenon that bypasses the individual self, or ego. The capacity to finesse genius can be learned, though often only through painful surrender, when the phoenix of genius arises out of the ashes of despair after a fruitless struggle with the unsolvable. Out of defeat comes victory; out of failure, success; and out of humbling, true self-esteem.

One of the problems in attempting to understand genius is that it takes near-genius to recognize it. The world frequently fails to identify genius altogether; society often gives acclaim to the work of genius without noting the intrinsic genius of its creation. Until one acknowledges the genius within oneself, one will have great difficulty recognizing it in others—we can only see without that which we realize within. In recent times, for example, Mikhail Gorbachev has been the subject of enormous worldwide attention, but the world did not really acknowledge his intrinsic *genius*. Single-handedly, in only a few short years, he completely revolutionized one of the greatest empires on Earth, and his only sources of power were his inspiration and vision. (Had the communist regime been based on power, nothing could have overturned it; because it was based on force, it was destined to come to an end under the hand of a charismatic leader aligned with power.)[5]

Genius is one of the greatest untapped resources of our society. It is no more specific than it is personal. People of great gifts not infrequently have multiple talents. A genius may be a genius in different realms and might have answers to a diversity of problems.

Society suffers a great loss because it does not know how to nurture its geniuses. They do not actually cost much to maintain—the source of genius is impersonal and true genius is seldom interested in money or fame. But society, in fact, is often either indifferent or hostile to genius.

The lifestyle of those whom we term genius is typically simple. Genius is characterized by an appreciation for resources and the economy of ingenuity, because the genius values life and sees the intrinsic worth of all its expressions. Inasmuch as time and resources are precious, doing more than is necessary is viewed as a waste; therefore, people of genius often lead very quiet lives and only reluctantly sally forth when there is a cause that must be supported. There is no need to "get" when you already "have." Genius, because it is in touch with an endless source of supply, experiences only a minimum of need. (Such simplicity seems a common characteristic of true success in general.) The basis of this non-materiality, this seeming naïveté, is a radical understanding of the nature of the universe itself: that which supports life is supported by life; survival is thus effortless, and giving and receiving are one and the same thing.

Genius is notoriously interpreted as unconventionality or eccentricity. It is true that persons of genius, because of their alignment with high-energy attractors, have a different perspective on life; therefore, things have a different significance for them. The genius is frequently inspired to intense activity by insights beyond our understanding.

Genius is not stardom. Those of genius who attain

prominence are a very small minority. There remains a legion of geniuses who achieve no such status; many appear in no way noteworthy and may, in fact, have never had formal higher education. What characterizes this type is the capacity to utilize exhaustively what experience they have, and to capitalize on it by the dedication necessary to reach a high degree of mastery. Many productive geniuses are not recognized until years after their death. In fact, the gift—or curse—of genius often brings about unfortunate consequences during an individual's earthly lifetime.

One characteristic of genius is the capacity for great intensity, which is often expressed in a cyclic form. When inspired, the person of genius may work twenty hours a day to realize a solution while it is still fresh in mind. These periods of intense activity are interspersed with intervals of apparent stasis that are in actuality intervals of fermentation, a necessary part of the creative process. Therefore, the personality of the genius sometimes seems to incorporate polar extremes. Geniuses understand the need for creating a space for ideas to crystallize. The stage is often set by complete distraction. Creativity occurs under appropriate inner, not outer circumstances. We all know stories of people who have gotten the answers to complex problems while sitting in traffic on the freeway.

A primary reason that so many people fail to recognize, and therefore empower, their own genius is because in the popular mind, genius is confused with a high IQ. This is a gross misunderstanding. It would be more helpful to see genius as simply an extraordinarily high degree of savvy in a given area of human activity.

The misconception about IQ has arisen from the fact that many celebrated geniuses in the fields of mathematics and physics indeed did have high IQs; however, in those fields, the IQ necessary to comprehend the work is a prerequisite. There are droves of non-cerebral artistic geniuses, musical geniuses, designers and inventors, geniuses in many fields whose talent is that of innovative creativity within specified areas.

Let us remember that IQ is merely a measure of academic capacity for logically comprehending symbols and words. The values that one lives by are more definitive of genius than IQ. From our studies, it appears that the alignment of one's goals and values with high-energy attractors is more closely associated with genius than anything else. Genius can be more accurately identified by perseverance, courage, concentration, enormous drive, and absolute integrity. Talent alone is not enough. Dedication of an unusual degree is required to achieve mastery, and in the simplest definition, one could say that genius is the capacity for an extraordinary degree of mastery in one's calling. A formula followed by all geniuses, prominent or not, is: Do what you like to do best, and do it to the very best of your ability.

CHAPTER 16

Surviving Success

The tragic careers of many individuals of genius subsequent to being discovered and celebrated by the public, illustrate that there is success, and then there is Success. The former frequently jeopardizes life, while the latter enhances it. True Success enlivens and supports the spirit; it has not to do with isolated attainments, but being successful as a total person, attaining a successful lifestyle that benefits not only yourself but everyone around you. Successful people's lives are empowered throughout by the context of their accomplishments.

In contradistinction, that which the tabloid world calls success often erodes the "successful" person's health and relationships; spiritual collapse is commonplace in the lives of the rich and famous. But what the world calls success is merely celebrity, and the capacity of celebrity to destroy is documented daily. Famous people constantly succumb to failed marriages, addiction, alcoholism, suicide, or untimely death. If we listed the names of all of the celebrities whose careers were blighted by such tragedies, it would fill a score of pages—the movie stars (Judy Garland, Marilyn Monroe, James Dean); the pop stars (Elvis Presley, Janis Joplin, Jimi Hendrix); the writers (Edgar Allan Poe, Jack London, Ernest Hemingway, F. Scott Fitzgerald)—the list goes on and on. In addition to such notorious examples of the price of celebrity are the uncounted thousands of less famous "successful" lives ruined by drug problems, or the twisting of personality whereby formerly decent folk become vain, cruel, self-centered, and inordinately self-indulgent.

It is not just that such people have gotten too much wealth, too much fame, or too much attention, but that these influences distorted their egos and reinforced what might be called the small self instead of the big Self. The small self is the part of us that is vulnerable to flattery; the big Self is an aspect of our more evolved nature, which is humble and grateful for success. The self aligns with weak attractor patterns; the Self is aligned with high power energy fields.

Whether it uplifts or destroys us depends not upon success itself, but on how it is integrated into our personalities. Whether we are proud or humble; whether we are egotistic or grateful; whether we deem ourselves better than others because of our talents or consider them a gift for which we are thankful—these are the determining factors. We all know people for whom even a bit of success is corrupting, who become arrogant, officious, and controlling when given a little authority. And we all know people of much greater authority who are cordial, sensitive, and caring.

When we come to know the powerful men of the world, captains of industry, presidents of banks, Nobel Prize winners, and members of legendary American families, it is striking to see how many are open, warm, sincere, and view success as a responsibility, noblesse oblige. These are truly successful people, notably courteous and considerate to all; whether visiting potentates or talking to servants, they treat everyone as an equal. The truly successful have no inclination to act arrogantly, because they consider themselves not better but more fortunate than others. They see their position as a stewardship, a responsibility to exercise their influence for the greatest benefit of all.

What allows the truly successful to be so gracious, open, and giving can be explained through our formula of causality:

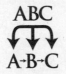

$$ABC$$
$$A \text{-} B \text{-} C$$

The truly successful identify with the ABC. They realize that they are a channel acted through to create success in the outer world. Inasmuch as they identify with the sources of success, they have no anxiety about losing it. But a person who views his success in the realm of the external, A→B→C, will always be insecure, because its source is thought to be "out there." Solid confidence comes from the knowledge that the source of success is within. By believing that the source of power lies outside oneself, one becomes powerless and vulnerable and, therefore, defensive and possessive. True success originates from within, independent of external circumstances.

The ladder of success seems to have three main steps. Initially, it is what we "have" that counts; status depends upon visible signs of material wealth. As one progresses, status is afforded by what one "does," rather than what one has. At this level on the ladder, one's position and activities bring significant social status, but the attraction of social roles loses glamour as one achieves mastery and matures; it is what one has accomplished that is important. Finally, one is concerned only with what one has become as a result of life's experiences. Such people have a charismatic "presence" that is the outer manifestation of the grace of their inner power. In their company, we feel the effect of the powerful attractor energy patterns with which they are aligned and which they reflect. Success comes as the automatic consequence of aligning one's life with high-power energy patterns.

Why is true success so relatively effortless? It might be likened to the magnetic field created by an electric current running through a wire. The higher the power of the current, the greater the magnetic field that it generates. And the magnetic field itself then influences everything in its presence. There are very few at the top. The world of the mediocre, however, is one of intense competition, and the bottom of the pyramid is crowded. Charismatic winners are sought out; losers have to strive to be accepted. People who are loving, kind, and thoughtful of others have more friends than they can count; success in every area of life is a reflex to those who are aligned with successful patterns. And the capacity to be able to discern the difference between the strong patterns of success and the weak patterns leading to failure is now available to each of us.

CHAPTER 17

Physical Health and Power

We become healthy, as well as wealthy, by being wise. But what is wisdom? According to our research, it is the result of alignment with high-power attractor patterns. Although in the average life we find a mixture of energy fields, the pattern with the highest power dominates. We have now explored sufficient material to be able to introduce a basic dictum of nonlinear dynamics and attractor research: *attractors create context*. In essence, this means that one's motive, which arises from the principles to which one is committed, determines one's capacity to understand and, thereby, gives significance to one's actions.

The effect of alignment with principle is nowhere more striking than in its physiologic consequences. Alignment with high-energy attractor patterns results in health; alignment with weak ones results in disease. This syndrome is specific and predictable. That high energy patterns can be proven to strengthen and low energy patterns to weaken through a demonstration meeting the scientific criterion of one-hundred-percent replicability is a fact with which the reader by now is thoroughly familiar.

The human central nervous system clearly has an exquisitely sensitive capacity to differentiate between life-supportive and life-destructive patterns. High-power attractor energy fields, which make the body go strong, release brain endorphins and have a tonic effect on all of the organs, whereas adverse stimuli release adrenaline, which suppresses immune response and instantaneously causes both weakness and enervation of specific organs, depending on the nature of the stimulus.

It is this type of phenomenon upon which treatment modalities such as chiropractic, acupuncture, reflexology, and many others are based. All of these treatments, however, are designed to correct the results of an energy imbalance, but unless the basic attitude that is causing the energy imbalance is corrected, the illness tends to return. People by the millions in self-help groups have demonstrated that health and recovery from the whole gamut of human behavioral problems and illnesses come as a consequence of adopting attitudes correlated with high-energy attractor patterns.

Generally speaking, physical and mental health are attendant upon positive attitudes, whereas ill health, both physical and mental, is associated with such negative attitudes as resentment, jealousy, hostility, self-pity, fear, anxiety, etc. In the field of psychoanalysis, positive attitudes are called welfare emotions, and the negative ones are called emergency emotions. Chronic immersion in emergency emotions results in physical or mental ill health and a gross weakening of one's personal power. How does one overcome negative attitudes so as to avoid this atrophy of power and health? Clinical observation indicates that the patient must reach a decision point. A sincere desire for change allows one to seek higher attractor energy patterns in their various expressions.

One does not get over pessimism by associating with cynics; the popular idea that you are defined by the company you keep has some clinical basis.

Attractor patterns tend to dominate any field in which they are received; thus, all that is really necessary is to expose oneself to a high-energy field and one's inner attitudes will spontaneously begin to change. This is a well-known phenomenon among self-help groups—as reflected in the saying, "Just bring the body to the meeting." If you merely expose yourself to the influence of higher patterns, they begin to "rub off"; as it is said, "You get it by osmosis."

It is generally held by traditional medicine that stress is the cause of many human disorders and illnesses. The problem with this diagnosis is that it does not accurately address the source of the stress. It looks to blame external circumstances, without realizing that *all stress is internally generated by one's attitudes*. It is not life's events, but one's reaction to them, that activates the symptoms of stress. A divorce, as we have said, can bring agony or relief. Challenges on the job can result in stimulation or anxiety, depending on whether one's supervisor is seen as a teacher or an ogre.

Our attitudes stem from our positions, and our positionality has to do with motive and therefore context. According to the overall way that we interpret the meaning of events, the same situation may be tragic or comic. Physiologically speaking, in the choice of attitude, one chooses between anabolic endorphins or catabolic adrenaline and stress hormones.

———

It would be foolish to claim that the only impacts on our health are those originating internally. Impersonal elements of the physical world can also increase or decrease our strength. Here, too, kinesiologic testing is valuable. It will clearly show that synthetics, plastics, artificial coloring, preservatives, insecticides, and artificial sweetener (just to mention a few) make the body go weak; whereas substances that are pure, organic, or made by human hands tend to make us go strong. If we experiment with vitamin C, for example, we find that organic vitamin C is superior to chemically produced ascorbic acid; the former makes you go strong and the latter does not. Eggs from organically fed free-range chickens have much more intrinsic power than eggs from caged and chemically fed chickens. The health-food movement seems to have been right all along.

Unfortunately, neither the American Medical Association nor the National Council on Food and Nutrition has a history of being enlightened in the field of nutrition. The scientific community now finally recognizes that nutrition is related to behavior and health, but this simple observation caused a controversy when Linus Pauling and I claimed, twenty years ago, in the book *Orthomolecular Psychiatry*, that nutrition affects the chemical environment of the brain and blood-stream, and thereby influences various behaviors, emotions, mental disorders, and brain chemistry.[1]

More recently, this author published a series of papers, the last in 1991, on a twenty-year study showing that a regimen of certain vitamins prevented the development of a neurological disorder called tardive dyskinesia, a frequently irreversible disorder that occurs in a high percentage of patients on long-term treatment with major anti-psychotics.[2] In a study of

61,000 patients, treated by 100 different doctors over a twenty-year period, the introduction of vitamins B3, C, E, and B6 decreased the expected rate of this terrible neurologic disorder from 25 percent to .04 percent.[3] (Among 61,000 patients protected by high-dosage vitamin therapy, only 37, rather than the predicted nearly 20,000, developed the disorder.)[4]

The paper was largely ignored in the United States because there was still no paradigm to give it credibility. The medical profession has simply been uninterested in nutrition, and organized medicine has traditionally been less than kind to innovators. It is helpful to remember that it is a foible of human nature to stoutly defend an established position despite overwhelming evidence against it; the only healthy way to deal with such lack of recognition is acceptance. Once we really understand the human condition, we will feel compassion where we once might have felt condemnation. Compassion is one of the highest of all of the energy attractor power patterns. As we shall see, our capacity to understand, forgive, and accept is directly linked to our personal health.

CHAPTER 18

Wellness and the Disease Process

It has been a common observation throughout the ages that certain diseases are associated with certain emotions and attitudes. The medieval concept of "melancholy," for instance, connected depression with impairment of the liver. In contemporary times, many physical disorders have been clearly linked with the emotions of stress.

That emotions do have physiologic consequences is well documented. In the early days of psychoanalysis, research to identify specific diseases with specific psychological conflicts gave rise to the whole field of psychosomatic medicine. We have all heard about the connection between heart disease and "type A" personalities versus "type B" personalities, and of how suppressed anger results in hypertension and strokes. The presumption has been that emotions affect hormonal change through neurotransmitter variations in different areas of the brain associated with controlling different organs by way of the sympathetic or autonomic nervous system.

In more recent years, concern over the spread of AIDS has given great impetus to research on the body's immune system. Generally, it appears that what is experienced as stress results in suppression of the thymus gland; with this, the body's defenses are impaired. But the various research approaches to this topic fail to examine the relationship between belief systems and attitudes, and the resultant context of perception that determines the nature of individual experience. The etiology of stress is always related to the organism's proclivity to respond to stimuli in specific and characteristic patterns. Drawing on what we already know from the mathematics of nonlinear dynamics and attractor research, as clinically confirmed by kinesiology and acupuncture, we can derive a formulation of the basic nature of the disease process itself.

An idea or constellation of thoughts presents itself in consciousness as an attitude that tends to persist over time; this attitude is associated with an attractor energy field of corresponding power or weakness. The result is a perception of the world creating events appropriate to trigger the specific emotion. All attitudes, thoughts, and beliefs are also connected with various pathways, called "meridians" of energy, to all of the body's organs. Through kinesiologic testing, it can be demonstrated that specific acupuncture points are linked with specific attitudes, and the meridian, in turn, serves as the energy channel to specific muscles and body organs.[1] These specific meridians have been traditionally named according to the organs that they energize; for instance, the heart meridian, gallbladder meridian, etc.[2]

There is nothing mysterious about these vital internal communications, and they can be demonstrated in seconds to anyone's satisfaction. As we know, if you hold a particular negative thought in mind, a very specific muscle will go weak; if you then replace the thought with a positive idea, the same muscle will instantly go strong.[3] The connection between mind and body is immediate, so the body's responses shift and change from instant to instant in response to one's train of thoughts and the associated emotions.

We have referred to the *law of sensitive depend-ence on initial conditions*, which draws upon the science of nonlinear dynamics and its associated math-ematics.[4] We will recall that this describes the manner in which a minuscule variation in a pattern of inputs can result in a very significant change in the eventual output. This is because the repetition of a slight variation over time results in a progressive change of pattern, or, sometimes, even a leap to a new harmon-ic when the increment increases logarithmically. The effect of the minute variation becomes amplified until it eventually affects the whole system and an entire new energy pattern evolves, which itself may, by the same process, then result in a further variation, and so on.

In the world of physics, this process is called "turbulence," and is the subject of an enormous amount of research, especially in the field of aerody-namics, in the combined focus of physics and mathe-matics. Such turbulence, when it occurs in the attractor energy fields of consciousness, creates an emotional upset that continues until a new level of homeostasis is established.

When the mind is dominated by a negative world-view, the direct result is a repetition of minute changes in energy flows to the various body organs. The subtle field of overall physiology is affected in all of its com-plex functions, mediated by electron transfer, neural hormonal balance, nutritional status, etc. Eventually, an accumulation of infinitesimal changes becomes discernible through measurement techniques, such as electron microscopy, magnetic imaging, x-ray, or biochemical analysis. But by the time these changes are detectable, the disease process is already well advanced in its own self-perpetuating resonances.

We could say that the invisible universe of thought and attitude becomes visible as a consequence of the body's habitual response. If we consider the millions of thoughts that go through the mind continuously, it is not surprising that the body's condition could radically change to reflect prevailing thought patterns, as modified by genetic and environmental factors.[5] It is the *persistence* and repetition of the stimulus that, through the law of sensitive dependence on initial conditions, results in the observable disease process. The stimulus that sets off the process may be so minute that it escapes detection itself.

If this scheme of disease formation is correct, then all disease should be reversible by changing thought patterns and habitual responses. In fact, spontaneous recoveries from every disease known to mankind have been recorded throughout history. (This phenomenon was the subject of the TV news show 20/20 on April 8, 1994.) Traditional medicine has documented spontaneous "cures," but has never had the conceptual tools with which to investigate the phenomenon. But even thoroughly modern surgeons are very reluctant to operate on anyone who is convinced that he will die during the surgery, because not infrequently such patients do just that.

It is said in Alcoholics Anonymous that there is no recovery until the subject experiences an essential change of personality.[6] This is the basic change first manifested by AA founder Bill W.—a profound transformation in total belief system, with a sudden leap in consciousness.[7] Such a major metamorphosis in attitude was first formally studied by the American psychiatrist Harry Tiebout, of Greenwich, Connecticut, who discovered it while treating a hopeless alcoholic woman named Marty M., the first woman in AA. She underwent a sudden change of personality to a degree unaccountable through any known therapeutic method. Dr. Tiebout documented that she was transformed from an angry, self-pitying, intolerant, and egocentric posture to a kind and gentle one, and became forgiving and loving. Her example is important because it so clearly demonstrates this key element in recovery from any progressive or hopeless disease. Dr. Tiebout wrote the first of a series of papers on this observation under the title "The Power of Surrender."[8]

In every studied case of recovery from hopeless and untreatable diseases, there has been this major shift in consciousness so that the attractor patterns that resulted in the pathologic process no longer dominated. The steps necessary for recovery from such grave illnesses were formalized by the first 100 alcoholics who recovered; these became the well-known 12 steps suggested by AA and all of the 12-step recovery groups that have followed.[9] The fact that pursuing these steps has resulted in the recovery of millions of people suggests that this experience may have a universal applicability to all disease processes. The advice Dr. Carl Jung gave Rowland H.—"Throw yourself wholeheartedly into any spiritual group that appeals to you, whether you believe in it or not, and hope that in your case a miracle may occur"[10]—may hold true for anyone who wishes to recover from a progressive disease.

In spontaneous recovery, there is frequently a marked increase in the capacity to love and the awareness of the importance of love as a healing factor and modality. We have been told by numerous books on the best-seller list that to love is to live healthily. But the mind resists change as a matter of pride. Love of our fellow man can ensue only when we stop condemning, fearing, and hating others. Such radical change can be disorienting; the courage to endure the temporary discomfort of growth is also required. Recovery from any disease process is dependent on willingness to explore new ways of looking at one's self and life. This includes the capacity to endure inner fears when belief systems are shaken. People cherish and cling to their hates and grievances; to heal humanity, it may be necessary to pry whole populations away from lifestyles of spite, attack, and revenge.

A prime difficulty with thoughts and behaviors associated with the energy fields that calibrate below 200 is that they cause counter-reactions. A familiar law of the observable universe is that force results in equal and opposite counterforce. All attacks, therefore, whether mental or physical, result in counterattack. Malice literally makes us sick; we are always the victims of our own spite. Even secret hostile thoughts result in a physiologic attack on one's own body.

On the other hand, like love, laughter heals because it arises through viewing a small context from a larger and more inclusive one, which removes the observer from the victim posture. Every joke reminds us that our reality is transcendent, beyond the specifics of events. Gallows humor, for instance, is based on the juxtaposition of the opposites of a paradox; the relief of basic anxiety then results in a laugh. One of the frequent accompaniments of sudden enlightening realizations is laughter. The cosmic joke is the side-by-side comparison of illusion with reality.

Humorlessness, in contrast, is inimical to health and happiness. Totalitarian systems are notably devoid of humor at every level. Laughter, which brings acceptance and freedom, is a threat to their rule through force and intimidation. It is hard to oppress people who have a good sense of humor. Beware the humorless, whether in a person, institution, or belief system; it is always accompanied by an impulse to control and dominate, even if its proclaimed objective is to create prosperity or peace.

One cannot create peace as such. Peace is the natural state of affairs when that which prevents it is removed. Relatively few people are genuinely committed to peace as a realistic goal. In their private lives, people prefer being "right" at whatever cost to their relationships or themselves. A self-justified positionality is the real enemy of peace. When solutions are sought on the level of coercion, no peaceful resolution is possible.

The healthcare field itself demonstrates how attempts to control only compound themselves into a burgeoning bureaucratic morass. Complexity is costly, and systems are as weak and inefficient as the attitudes that underlie their construction. Systems associated with very weak attractor fields are ineffective because of their inherent dishonesty and become wasteful and cumbersome. The healthcare industry is so overburdened with fear and regulation that it can barely function. Healing from individual illness (or the healing of the health-care industry itself) can only occur by the progressive steps of elevation of motive and abandonment of self-deception, to attain a new clarity of vision. There are not any villains; the fault is in the misalignment of the system itself.

If we say that health, effectuality, and prosperity are the natural states of being in harmony with reality, then anything less than that calls for internal scrutiny rather than the projection of blame on things outside of the system itself. Attractor patterns obey the laws of their own physics, even if they are not Newtonian; to forgive is to be forgiven. As we have observed repeatedly, in a universe where everything is connected with everything else, there is no such thing as an "accident," and nothing is outside of the universe. Because the power of the actual elements is unseen and only the manifestation of effects is observable, there is an illusion of "accidental" events. A sudden and unexpected event may appear to be random, unrelated to observable causes, but its actual origin can be traced through research. A sudden illness always has discernible antecedents; even accident-proneness involves numerous small preparatory steps before the so-called "accidents" occur.

A disease process is evidence that something is amiss in the workings of the mind, and that is where the power to effect a change resides. Treating an illness as a physical process only, within the A→B→C illusionary world of effects, does not correct the origin of the dysfunction, and is palliative rather than curative. It is possible for a lifelong affliction to heal rapidly with a mere shift of attitude; but although this shift may seem to occur in a split second, it may take years of inner advance preparation.

We remember that the critical point in any complex system is the locus at which the least power is required to alter the whole system. A move of even one pawn on the chessboard completely changes the possibilities of the game. Every detail of the belief system that we hold has consequences for better or for worse. It is for this reason that there is no condition that is incurable or hopeless; somewhere, sometime, somebody has recovered from it through the processes that we have described.

It is instrumental not only in recovery, but for any major advancement of consciousness to have compassion for oneself and all of mankind as we go through the painful struggles of evolution. Only thus do we become healers as well as healed. And only thus may we hope to be healed of any malaise, physical or spiritual.

Does all of this mean that if we learn to operate on the level of unconditional love, we will become immortal? No. The protoplasm of the physical body is vulnerable to its own genetic programming, as well as to its external environment. But from the viewpoint of consciousness level 500 and above, it appears that death itself is only an illusion, and that life goes on unimpeded by the limitation of perception which results from being localized in a physical body. Consciousness is the vital energy that both gives life to the body and survives beyond the body in a different realm of existence.

PART THREE:
MEANING

CHAPTER 19

The Database of Consciousness

The great Swiss psychoanalyst Carl Jung, noting the ubiquity of archetypal patterns and symbols, deduced the "collective unconscious," a bottomless, subconscious pool of all the shared experiences of the whole human race.[1] We may think of it as a vast, hidden database of human awareness, characterized by powerful, universal organizing patterns. Such a database, comprising all of the information ever available to human consciousness, implies stunning inherent capabilities; it is far more than just a giant storehouse of information awaiting a retrieval process. Tapping into all that has ever been experienced anywhere in time, the great promise of the database is its capacity to "know" virtually anything the moment it is "asked."

This is the origin of all information obtained sub- or supra-rationally, by intuition or premonition, by divination or dreams, or by "lucky" guess. It is the fountainhead of genius, the well of inspiration, and the source of "uncanny" psychic knowledge, including "foreknowledge." It is, of course, the inventory drawn upon by kinesiologic testing. Thinkers who are troubled by the notion of "paranormal" or non-rational knowledge usually balk at logical—or illogical—inconsistencies with Newtonian concepts of simultaneity, causality, or time and space.

In actuality, it is a bigger universe than that. These same thinkers will scan the evening sky and find pleasure in identifying a favorite constellation. But in reality, there are no such things as constellations. That familiar pattern of "stars" is made up of points of light originating from totally unrelated sources—some millions of light-years closer or farther away; some even in different galaxies; some actually separate galaxies themselves; and many have, millennia since, burnt out and ceased to "exist." Those lights have no spatial or temporal relationship. It is not only the shape of a dipper or bear or man, but only the very pattern, the "constellation" itself, that is projected onto the sky by the eye of the beholder. Yet the zodiac is still "real" because we conceive it, in the first sense of the word. Astrology still "exists," and for many people is quite a useful pragmatic tool in explaining themselves and their relationships. Why not? The database of consciousness is an infinite resource.

The database behaves like an electrostatic condenser with a field of potentiality, rather than like a battery with a stored charge. A question cannot be asked unless there is already the potentiality of an answer. The reason for this is that both the question and answer are created out of the same paradigm and, therefore, are exactly concordant. There is no "up" without an already existent "down." Causality occurs as simultaneity rather than as sequence; synchronicity is the term used by Dr. Jung to explain this phenomenon in human experience.[2] As we understand from our examination of advanced physics, an event "here" in the universe does not "cause" an event "there" in the universe. Instead, both appear simultaneously, and the sequence is that of observation itself.

What is the connection between these events, then, if it is not a Newtonian linear sequence of cause and effect? Obviously, the two events are related or connected to each other in some invisible manner, but not by gravity or magnetism, or a cosmic wind or an ether; they are encompassed by an attractor field of such magnitude that it includes both events. We may know this is so because otherwise the events would not be observable as events at all, much less simultaneously or as related to each other in time or supposed causality.

The "connection" between these two events occurs only in the observer's consciousness—he "sees" a connection and describes a "pair" of events, hypothesizing a relationship. This relationship is a concept that exists solely in the mind of the observer; it is not necessary that any corollary external event exist in the universe. Unless there is an underlying attractor pattern, nothing can be experienced. Thus, the entire manifest universe is its own simultaneous expression and experience of itself.

Omniscience is omnipotent and omnipresent. There is no distance between the unknown and the known. The known is manifested from the unknown merely by the asking. The Empire State Building was born in the mind of its architect. Human consciousness is the agent whereby an unseen concept is transformed into its manifest experience, such as "that building," and thus frozen in time. What actually "happened" at the intersection of West 34th Street and Fifth Avenue in New York City in 1931 is still there for all to see. What "happened" in the consciousness of its creators also stands recorded in the database for all of us to see. Both exist complete, but in different sensory domains. By transferring concept into concrete and steel, the architect simply enabled the rest of us to experience his own inner vision.

We supposedly "normal" humans are completely preoccupied with our function as transformers of concepts from the invisible level, ABC, to the sensory perceptual level of A→B→C. Extraordinary individuals live primarily in the world of the ABC. (Those who live beyond that, in the completely formless domain of pure consciousness itself, we call mystics.) To such individuals, the origin of everything is obvious; they are uninterested in the process of making things visible and manifest. In everyday life, these are the creative people who spawn new enterprises and then turn over their execution and management to others. The yet more advanced—mystics—conclude that only their inner ABC level of awareness is "real" and that the observable world is a dream or illusion. It should be pointed out, however, that this is only another limited point of view. There is neither real nor non-real, only that which *is*. That which is, is so, from all viewpoints or none.

Existence without form is not really imaginable, yet at the same time it is the ultimate reality. This includes both yin and yang, the unmanifest and the manifest, the formed and the formless, the seen and the unseen, the temporal and the timeless. Thus, the seeming real world is simultaneously the *Real* world, for that which is All Possibility must include within it all that is. Creation is, therefore, continuous, or there could be no creation at all. To look for the "beginning" of creation is to proceed from an artificial notion of time. The "start" of something that is outside of time cannot be located in time. The "big bang" can only occur in the mind of an observer.

The universe is very cooperative. Inasmuch as the universe is not different from consciousness itself, it is happy to create whatever we wish to find "out there." The problem is with the concept of cause itself, which begs the question by presuming a time warp, a sequence, or a string of events that would make sense. If we step outside of time, there are no causes at all. We could say that the manifest world originates out of the unmanifest, but that again would be inferring a sequential causal series in time—that is, unmanifest becoming manifest. Once beyond the warp of time, with its implicit restrictions of comprehension to terms of mere sequence, there is no backwards or forwards. It is then just as valid to say, reciprocally, that the manifest universe causes the unmanifest; and at a certain level of understanding, this is demonstrably true. If, for example, we look at electrons lined up on one side of a dielectric membrane and protons lined up on the other side in an equal balance, how can we say which side causes the other to line up? Similarly, though healing is a consequence of compassion, compassion is not its "cause." In an energy field of 600 or higher, almost anything has a tendency to heal.

The source of all life and all form is, of necessity, greater than its manifestations; yet, it is neither different from them nor separate to any degree. There is no conceptual artifact of separation between creator and created. As scripture states, that which is, was, and always shall be.

Time, then, is a locus of the perception of a hologram that already stands complete; it is a subjective, sensory effect of a progressively moving point of view. There is no beginning or end to a hologram. It is already everywhere, complete. In fact, the appearance of being "unfinished" is part of its completeness. Even the phenomenon of "unfoldment" itself reflects a limited point of view. There is in reality no enfolded versus unfolded universe; there is actually only a becoming awareness. Our perception of events happening in time is analogous to a traveler watching the landscape unfold before him. But to say that the landscape unfolds before the traveler is merely a figure of speech. Nothing is actually unfolding; nothing is actually becoming manifest. There is only the progression of awareness.

These paradoxes dissolve in the greater paradigm that includes both opposites, wherein opposites as such are only the actual location of the observer. This transcendence of opposition occurs spontaneously at consciousness levels of 600 and above. The notion that there is a "knower" verses a "known" is in itself dualistic, in that it implies a separation between subject and object (which, again, can only be inferred by the artificial adoption of an arbitrary point of observation). The Maker of all things in heaven and on earth, of all things visible and invisible, stands beyond both, includes both, and is one with both. Existence is, therefore, merely a statement that awareness is aware of its awareness and of its expression as consciousness.

Ontology need not be speculative. It is, after all, only the theology of existence; anyone who is aware that he exists already has access to its highest formulations and beyond. There is only one absolute truth; all the rest are semi-facts spawned from the artifacts of limited perception and positionality. "To be or not to be" is not a choice; one may decide to be this or that, but to *be* is, simply, the only fact there is.

All of the foregoing has been expressed at various times in man's intellectual history by sages who have moved beyond duality in their awareness. But even then, to claim that the comprehension of the non-duality of existence is superior to its realization as dual is again to fall into another illusion. There is, ultimately, neither duality nor non-duality; there is only awareness. Only awareness itself can state that it is beyond all concepts such as "is" or "is not." This must be so, because "is" can be conceived only by consciousness itself.

Awareness itself is beyond even consciousness. Therefore, it may be said that the Absolute is unknowable exactly because it is beyond knowing, because it is beyond the reach of consciousness itself. Those who have attained such a state of awareness report that it cannot be described and can have no meaning for anyone without the experience of that context. Nonetheless, this is the true state of Reality, universally and eternally; we merely fail to recognize it. Such a recognition is the essence of enlightenment and the final resolution of the evolution of consciousness to the point of self-transcendence.[3]

CHAPTER 20

The Evolution of Consciousness

Thousands of calculations and innumerable calibrations drawn from kinesiologic testing of individuals and from historical analysis indicate that the average advance in the level of consciousness throughout the global population is on the average little more than five points for a lifetime. Apparently, from untold millions of individual experiences in one's life, usually only a few lessons are ever really learned. The attainment of wisdom is apparently slow and painful, and few are willing to relinquish familiar, even if inaccurate, views; resistance to change or growth is considerable. It would seem that most people are willing to die rather than alter those belief systems that confine them to lower levels of consciousness.

If this is true, then what is the prognosis for the human condition? Is a five-point advance per generation all that can be expected? This troubling question deserves our attention.

In the first place, as we can observe from the distribution of levels of consciousness throughout the world population, great masses of our species are at the low end of the evolutionary scale, and still rely on force to compensate for their actual powerlessness. More advanced cultures exhibit more variation. The Japanese capitalized on the lessons of World War II and collectively made a major jump in their evolution. On the other hand, America's level of consciousness sank as a result of the Vietnam War; what was actually learned as yet remains to be seen.

Unfortunately, our entertainment in general trades

on emotional sensationalism, and so gravitates toward violence. Murder is nightly family fare on television; our children grow up on a steady mental diet of it. Americans have learned to enjoy the gruesome—and the more bizarre, the better. Cruelty and havoc are becoming status quo. In the city of Phoenix, where an initiative requiring children to have parental permission to carry guns recently failed, ABC news on January 1, 1993, reported the handgun killing of a two-and-a-half-year-old by a three-year-old. It seems that society institutionalizes certain self-propagating levels of consciousness that become an ingrained characteristic of various social strata.

Nonetheless, there remains free choice and thus a considerable potential for individual mobility and variety of experience, making available alternate options. From our study of advanced theoretical physics, nonlinear dynamics, and the nature of nonlinear equations, it is clear that, at least in theory, choice is not only possible, but inevitable. It is out of regularity that irregularity appears; all attractor patterns are connected to each other, if only by a single "strand," so to speak. But how exactly do transformational choices occur? What occasions them? Who makes them and why? This is a crucial subject regarding which few principles have been defined.

Growth and development are irregular and nonlinear. Practically nothing is known about the essential nature of growth, or any "process" in nature for that matter. No one has ever studied the nature of life itself, only its images and consequences. There simply has not been an adequate mathematics to comprehend it; linear differential equations brought us to approximations, but not to essence. A simple sprouting seed performs incredible wonders through an intrinsic wizardry of which we have no understanding whatsoever.

As is commonly observed, growth, both individual and collective, can take place either slowly or suddenly. It is not limited by restraints, but by tendencies. Innumerable options are open to everyone all the time, because people want the context that would make them attractive. One's range of choice is ordinarily limited by one's vision.

Context, value, and meaning are merely different terms for a subtle web of energy patterns within an overall organizing attractor energy field—which is itself only part of a still larger one, and so on, in an infinite continuum throughout the universe, eventually including the total field of consciousness itself. While the sheer magnitude of such a complex of energy patterns seems beyond human cognizance, its totality is nonetheless comprehended by individuals whose consciousness reaches the 600 to 700 range. This gives us some idea of the enormous capacity for understanding possessed by those with advanced consciousness.

The most important element in facilitating an upward movement in consciousness is an attitude of willingness, which opens up the mind through new means of appraisal to the possible validity of new hypotheses. Although motives for change are as multitudinous as the innumerable facets of the human condition, they are most often found to arise spontaneously when the mind is challenged in the face of a puzzle or a paradox. Deliberately creating such an impasse is a customary device in certain disciplines, such as Zen, to finesse a leap of awareness.

On our scale of consciousness, there are two critical fulcrums that allow for major advancement. The first is at level 200, the initial level of empowerment. Here arises the willingness to stop blaming and accept responsibility for one's own actions, feelings, and beliefs. So long as cause and responsibility are projected outside of oneself, one must remain in the powerless mode of victimhood. The second is at the 500 level, reached by accepting love and nonjudgmental forgiveness as a lifestyle, exercising unconditional kindness to all persons, things, and events without exception. (In 12-step recovery groups, it is said that there is no such thing as a justified resentment. Even if somebody "did you wrong," you are still free to choose your response and let the resentment go.) Once one makes this commitment, they begin to experience a different, more benign world as their perceptions evolve.

It is initially very challenging to understand that attitudes can alter the world one experiences and that there are numerous valid ways of experiencing it. But, as in viewing a hologram, what you see depends completely on the position from which you view it. Which position, then, is so-called "reality"?

In fact, *this is a holographic universe*. Each point of view reflects a position defined by the viewer's unique level of consciousness. If you are on this side of the hologram, your perception will hardly agree with that of the observer on the other side. "He must be crazy!" is a common reaction to such wide discrepancy. And the world is a set of holograms in limitless dimensions, not, as is often said, of mirrors—which are fixed in time and place and offer only a single reflection. Auditory experience also is part of a holographic series of attractor fields of all the sounds that ever were. The physical world is tactile, too. It has texture, color, dimension, and spatial relationships such as position and shape. Each of these is, again, part of an underlying sequence that, with all of the other qualities, goes back in to the "end of time" to the original source of its existence, which is *now*.

A hologram, we might say, is in and of itself a process. There is nothing fixed in a three-dimensional hologram. And what then of a four-dimensional hologram? It would include all possible instances of itself simultaneously. To change seems to be to move through time, but if time itself is transcended, then there is no such thing as sequence. If all is now, there is nothing to follow from here to there. Each hologram is in itself an evolutionary projection from an endless nonlinear matrix of events that are not causally related, but instead synchronous. Then, at the perceptual level of 600 to 700, what was, what is, and what will be are comprehended wordlessly within the complete, simultaneous holographic possibility.[1] The term "ineffable" here begins to take on meaning.

———

Let us attempt to better understand all of this through an example. Imagine a so-called "bum" on a street corner:

In a fashionable neighborhood in a big city stands

an old man in tattered clothes, alone, leaning against the corner of an elegant brownstone. Look at him from the perspective of various levels of consciousness, and note the differences in how he appears.

From the bottom of the scale, at a level of 20 (Shame), the bum is dirty, disgusting, and disgraceful. From level 30 (Guilt), he would be blamed for his condition. He deserves what he gets; he is probably a lazy welfare cheat. At 50 (Hopelessness), his plight might appear desperate, evidence that society cannot do anything about homelessness. At 75 (Grief), the old man looks tragic, friendless, and forlorn.

At a consciousness level of 100 (Fear), we might see the bum as threatening, a social menace. Perhaps we should call the police before he commits some crime. At 125 (Desire), he might represent a frustrating problem—why does somebody not do something? At 150 (Anger), the old man might look like he could be violent; or, on the other hand, one could be furious that such a condition exists. At 175 (Pride), he could be seen as an embarrassment or as lacking the self-respect to better himself. At 200 (Courage), we might be motivated to wonder if there is a local homeless shelter; all he needs is a job and a place to live.

At 250 (Neutrality), the bum looks okay, maybe even interesting. "Live and let live," we might say; after all, he is not hurting anyone. At 310 (Willingness), we might decide to go down there and see what we can do to cheer him up, or volunteer some time at the local mission. At 350 (Acceptance), the man on the corner appears intriguing. He probably has an interesting story to tell; he is where he is for reasons we may never understand. At 400 (Reason), he is a symptom of the current economic and social malaise, or perhaps a good subject for an in-depth psychological study, worthy of a government grant.

At the higher levels, the old man begins to look not only interesting, but friendly and even lovable. Perhaps we would then be able to see that he was, in fact, one who had transcended social limits and gone free, a joyful old guy with the wisdom of age in his face and the serenity that comes from indifference to material things. At level 600 (Peace), he is revealed as our own inner self in its temporary expression.

When approached, the bum's response to these different levels of consciousness would also vary. With some people, he would feel secure, with others, frightened or dejected. Some would make him angry, and others would delight him. Some people he would therefore avoid, and others greet with pleasure. (Thus it is said that what we meet is actually a mirror.)[2]

So much for the manner in which our level of consciousness decides what we see. It is equally true that having placed that construct upon the reality before us, we will react to it in a fashion predicted by the level from which we observe. External events may define conditions, but they do not determine the consciousness level of human response. We can take the more literal scene of our current penal system as an illustration.

Placed in an identical and extremely stressful environment, different inmates react in ways that vary extraordinarily according to their level of consciousness. Prisoners whose consciousness is at the lowest end of the scale sometimes attempt suicide. Others become psychotic, and some become delusional. Some in the same circumstances fall into despondency, go mute, and stop eating. Still others sit with head in hands, trying to hide tears of grief. A very frequent experience is that of fear, including paranoid defensiveness. In the same cellblock, we see other prisoners with a greater degree of energy going to rage, violent and assaultive and homicidal. Pride is everywhere present, in the form of macho bragging and struggles for dominance.

By contrast, some inmates find the courage to face the truth of why they are there, and begin to look at their own inner lives honestly. There are always some who just "roll with the punches" and try to get some reading done. At the level of Acceptance, we see prisoners who seek out help and join support groups. It is not unusual for an occasional inmate to take a new interest in learning, start studying in the prison library, or become a jailhouse lawyer (some of history's most influential political books were written behind bars). A few prisoners go through a transformation of consciousness and become loving and generous caregivers to their fellows. And it is not unheard of for a prisoner aligned with higher energy fields to become deeply spiritual, even to actively pursue enlightenment.

How we react depends upon the world we seem to be reacting to. Who we become, as well as what we see, are both determined by perception, which can be said, simply, to create the perceptual, experiential world. It is interesting to note that the further down the scale of consciousness a person is, the harder it is for them to maintain eye contact. At the low end, visual contact is avoided altogether. In contrast, as we go up the scale, the ability to hold a prolonged, and finally almost endless, gaze at great depth becomes characteristic. We are all familiar with the guarded glance of guilt, the glare of hostility, and, in contrast, the unblinking open-eyed-ness of innocence. *Power and perception go hand in hand*.

How, then, does perception work? What are its mechanics? That perception is subjectively unique is evidenced by common observation. We are all familiar with the example of a mock trial in law school, wherein different witnesses relate wildly divergent accounts of the same event. The mechanism of perception is like a movie theater in which the projector is consciousness itself. The forms on the film emulsion are the attractor energy patterns, and the moving pictures on the screen are the world that we perceive and call "reality." We could say that the configurations on the film are the ABC attractor fields in the mind, and the moving pictures on the screen are the A→B→C, which is observed as the phenomenal world.

This schema provides a model for a better understanding of the nature of causality, which occurs on the level of the film, but not on the level of the screen. Because the world routinely applies its efforts to the screen of life at the level of A→B→C, these endeavors are ineffectual and costly. Causality stems from the attractor patterns of levels of energy, the ABCs of the configurations imprinted on the film of mind, which are then illuminated by the light of consciousness.

The nature of the stream of consciousness, its

patterns of thought, perception, feeling, and memory, are the consequence of entrainment of the attractor energy field by which it is dominated. It is well to remember that *this domination is volitional*. It is not imposed, but is the outcome of one's own choices, beliefs, and goals.

By consent we synchronize with a field pattern that implies specific styles of processing and influences all our decisions according to its accompanying set of values and meanings. What appears as important and exciting from the perspective of one level might be boring or even repulsive at another level; truth is subjective. That fact can be seen as frightening. The current elevation of science to the status of infallible oracle is an expression of our insecure compulsion to feel that there is some kind of a measurable, universally predictable, objective world "out there" upon which we can truly rely.

But in transcending the emotional distortions of perception, science itself creates yet another conceptual distortion due to the limitation of its parameters. Science must of necessity remove data from context in order to study it, but in the end, it is only the context that gives the data its whole significance, value, or meaning. The eventual discovery arrived at by advanced theoretical physics can be reached from any organized field of human knowledge. The more detailed one's analysis of the structure of what is supposedly "out there," the more one discovers that what one is examining is, in fact, the nature of the intricate processes of consciousness which are actually originating from within. There is actually nothing "out there," other than consciousness itself. The habitual tendency to believe otherwise is a fundamental illusion, a vanity of the human mind, which tends always to view its transitory subject as "mine."

Objectively, it can be seen that thoughts really belong to the consciousness of the world; the individual mind merely processes them in new combinations and permutations. What seem to be truly original thoughts appear only through the medium of genius and are invariably felt by their authors to be found or given, not created. It may be the case that we are each unique, as no two snowflakes are alike; however, we are still just snowflakes.

We all inherit the human condition of mind in our seemingly unasked-for birth. To transcend the limitations of the mind, it is necessary to dethrone it from its tyranny as sole arbiter of reality. The mind's vanity confers its imprimatur of authenticity on the movie of life that it happens to view; the mind's very nature is to convince us that its unique view of experience is the genuine article. Each individual secretly feels that their experience of the world is the only true and accurate one.

In our discussion of the levels of consciousness, we noted that one of the downsides of Pride is denial. Every mind engages in denial in order to protect its supposed "correctness." This begets the fixity and resistance to change that prevents the average consciousness from advancing much more than five points in a lifetime. Great leaps in level of consciousness are always preceded by surrender of the illusion that "I know." Frequently, the only way one can reach this willingness to change is when one "hits bottom," that is, by running out a course of action to its end in the defeat of a futile belief system. Light cannot enter a closed box; the upside of catastrophe can be an opening to a higher level of awareness. If life is viewed as a teacher, it then becomes just that. Unless the painful lessons of life with which we deal are transformed through humility into gateways of growth and development, they are wasted.

We witness, we observe, we record apparent processions of experiences. But even in awareness itself, nothing actually happens. Awareness merely registers what is being experienced; it has no effect on it. Awareness is the all-encompassing attractor field of unlimited power identical with life itself. *There is nothing the mind believes that is not fallacious at a higher level of awareness.*

The mind identifies with its content. It takes credit and blame for what it believes, for it would be humbling to the mind's vanity to admit that the only thing it is doing is experiencing, and, in fact, it is only *experiencing experiencing* itself. The mind does not even experience the world, but only sensory reports of it. Even brilliant thoughts and deepest feelings are only experiences; ultimately, we have but one function: to experience experiencing.

The major limitation of consciousness is its innocence. Consciousness is gullible; it believes everything it hears. Consciousness is like hardware that will play back any software you put into it. We never lose the innate innocence of our own consciousness; it persists, naïve and trusting, like an impressionable child. Its only guardian is a discerning awareness that scrutinizes the incoming program.

Over the ages, it has been noted that merely observing the mind tends to increase one's level of consciousness.[3] A mind that is being watched becomes more humble and begins to relinquish its claims to omniscience. A growth in awareness can then take place. With humility comes the capacity to laugh at oneself and increasingly to be less the victim of the mind and more its master, as demonstrated by the famous Zen ox-herding pictures.

From thinking that we "are" our minds, we begin to see that we "have" minds, and that it is the mind that has thoughts, beliefs, feelings, and opinions. Eventually, we may arrive at the insight that all our thoughts are merely borrowed from the great database of consciousness and were never really our own to begin with. Prevailing thought systems are received, absorbed, identified with, and, in due time, replaced by new ideas that have become fashionable. As we place less value on such passing notions, they lose their capacity to dominate us, and we experience progressive freedom of, as well as from, the mind. This, in turn, ripens into a new source of pleasure; fittingly, the pleasure of existence itself matures as one ascends the scale of consciousness.

CHAPTER 21

The Study of Pure Consciousness

Various aspects of consciousness have been the subjects of traditional philosophy, and the expressions of consciousness as mind or emotion have been the subjects of the clinical sciences, but the nature of consciousness itself has never been clinically studied in any comprehensive sense.

In medicine, the presumption that consciousness is no more than a function of the brain is reflected in such statements as, "The patient regained consciousness." This routine, narrow depiction has assumed that consciousness is a mundane physical phenomenon, a self-evident priority for experience about which nothing more need to be said.

The one recurrent focus of interest on the subject has been speculation regarding what happens to man's consciousness at death. Does the power of life and awareness arise from a physical basis? Does the body sustain conscious life, or is it the other way around—the power of life sustains the body? Because the way the question is asked will be defined by the questioner's preconception of causality, the level of the questioner will predetermine the nature of the answer. Each questioner will therefore derive an answer representative of what is actually merely their own level of consciousness.

To the materialistic scientist, the question will appear nonsensical and a fruitless exercise in tautology. To those at the other pole (the "enlightened"), the question will seem comical, and the limited perception it reveals will elicit compassion. The common man might take on faith the authority of either, or of conventional religious teachings, to answer the question.

All discussions of life, death, and the final fate of consciousness must necessarily reflect differences of context. The reciprocal of René Descartes's famous phrase, "I think, therefore I am," is "I am, therefore I think." Because thinking takes place as form, Descartes is correct; that which has form must already have existence in order to have form. "I am" is a statement of awareness, witnessing that the capacity for experience is independent of form.[1] Descartes implies that consciousness is only aware of itself when it assumes form. But the enlightened throughout history have disagreed, customarily stating that consciousness is beyond form and is, indeed, the very omnipotent matrix out of which form arises. Modern physicists concur, for example David Bohm's concept of an "enfolded" versus an "unfolded" universe.

Without consciousness, there would be nothing to experience form. It could also be said that form itself, as a product of perception with no independent existence, is thus transitory and limited, whereas consciousness is all-encompassing and unlimited. How could that which is transitory, with a clear beginning and ending, create that which is formless, all-encompassing and omnipresent? However, if we see that the notion of limitation itself is merely a product of perception with no intrinsic reality, then the riddle solves itself: form becomes an expression of the formless. Ontologically, consciousness is an aspect of "Is-ness" and "Being-ness" and is implicit in man's definition of himself as human. Humanness is only one expression of beingness.

The operation of consciousness in human beings is the greater subject of our study. Although consciousness itself may be intangible, it is intrinsic to all human behavior. For purposes of this work, the problem is how to clinically explicate the connection between consciousness and behavior in an accurate, meaningful way that can be scientifically studied and validated. Fortunately, kinesiology categorically demonstrates the physical expression of sentience through the instantaneous reaction of the body to events experienced within consciousness. The technique affords us an elegant methodology, with an unmistakably established end point that can be calibrated, documented, and reproduced experimentally.

Characteristics of Pure Consciousness

Our vision of consciousness is linked with our concept of self: the more limited the sense of self, the smaller is the parameter of experiencing. Restricted paradigms of reality are global in their effects. As an example, our studies of the so-called "poor" have made it evident that "poorness" is not just a financial condition, but that the really "poor" are poor in all areas of life: poor in friendships, poor in verbal skills, poor in education, poor in social amenities, poor in resources, poor in health, and poor in overall level of happiness. Poorness, then, can be seen as a quality characteristic of a limited self-image resulting in a paucity of resources.[2] It is not a financial condition, but a level of consciousness. The energy of that level of awareness calibrates at about 60.

The identification and therefore experience of self could be limited to an identification of oneself as merely one's physical body. Then, of course, we might well ask: How does one then know that one has a physical body? Through observation, we note that the presence of the physical body is registered by the senses. The question follows—What is it then that is aware of the senses? How do we experience what the senses are reporting? Something greater, something more encompassing than the physical body, has to exist in order to experience that which is lesser; that something is mind itself. A person identifies with his body because his mind is experiencing the body. Patients who have lost sizable portions of their bodies report that their sense of self remains undiminished; such a person will say, "I'm still just as much me as I ever was."

The question then arises: How does one know what is being experienced by the mind? By observation and introspection, one can witness that thoughts have no capacity to experience themselves, but that something both beyond and more basic than thought experiences the sequence of thoughts, and that its sense of identity is unaltered by the content of the thoughts.

What is it that observes and is aware of all of the subjective and objective phenomena of life? It is consciousness itself that is both awareness and the source of experiencing. Both are purely subjective. Consciousness itself is not determined by content; thoughts flowing through consciousness are like fish swimming in the ocean. The ocean's existence is independent of the fish; the content of the sea does not define the nature of the water. Like a colorless ray, consciousness illuminates the object witnessed—thus its traditional depiction throughout world literature is with "light."[3]

Identification solely with the content of consciousness accounts for the experience of self as limited. In contrast, to identify with consciousness itself is to know that one's actual self is unlimited. When circumscribed self-identifications have been surmounted so that the sense of self is identified as consciousness itself, the condition is called "enlightened."[4]

One characteristic of the experience of pure consciousness is a perception of timelessness (or timelessness of perception). Consciousness is experienced as beyond all form and time and seen as everywhere equally present. It is described as "Is-ness" or "Being-ness" and, in the spiritual literature, "I-am-ness."[5] Consciousness does not recognize separation, which is the consequence of a limitation of perception. The enlightened state is of a "Oneness" in which there is no division into separate parts. Such division is only apparent from a localized perception; it is really only incidental to a fixed point of view.

Similar descriptions throughout the history of thought are in accord with the studies of William James, as reported in the Gifford lectures and the famous book *Varieties of Religious Experience*. The experience of consciousness itself has been described as rare, unique, ineffable, and "beyond mind;" as a thought-free state of Knowingness that is complete, all-inclusive, with neither need nor want, and beyond the limitation of experiencing a merely personalized, individual self.[6]

Another attribute of pure consciousness is cessation of the ordinary flow of thought or feeling. There is also a condition of the presence of infinite power, infinite compassion, gentleness, and love. In this state, the personal self becomes the Infinite Self. There is an accompanying recognition of the very origin of the capacity to experience self as Self. This awareness of self as Self is the culmination of the process of eliminating limited identifications.[7]

The steps necessary to be taken to facilitate awareness of the Self as consciousness have been well detailed historically. Numerous techniques have been prescribed to facilitate the removal of obstacles to expanded awareness; these can be found in the practice of various spiritual disciplines. The one process common to all such teachings is the progressive elimination of the identification of self as finite.[8]

Enlightenment is said to be relatively rare, not so much because of the difficulty of following the necessary steps, but because it is a condition of interest to very few, particularly in modern society. If we were to stop one thousand people on the street and ask them, "What is your greatest ambition in life?" how many would say, "To become enlightened"?

Contemporary Recognition of Higher Consciousness
The growing level of interest in consciousness as a scientific subject was evidenced by the first international conference on the subject, titled "Toward a Scientific Basis of Consciousness," held at the University of Arizona Health Sciences Center in Tucson, Arizona, on

April 12-17, 1994. This was an international, inter-disciplinary convocation of impressively credentialed scholars. However, among the numerous eminent presenters and the wide range of highly specialized subjects dealt with, there was little inquiry beyond rational/materialistic explanations of consciousness as a purely physical phenomenon (materialistic reductionism).

In fact, approaches to the subject of consciousness are as varied as human experience itself. We have cited many of the cutting-edge insights of modern inquiry into this issue in passing. It may be helpful to review the evolution of contemporary thought on this matter in order to proceed more clearly to our own conclusions.

The presence of some variety of consciousness is ordinarily considered to be the distinguishing characteristic of that which is living as opposed to that which is non-living. Life is the expression of consciousness in the observable or experiential world of form. But the totality of human experience attests that consciousness is both manifest and unmanifest. The awareness of consciousness within form is common; the awareness of pure consciousness, beyond form, is exceptional.

This "experience" of pure consciousness itself, devoid of all content, has been consistently reported throughout human history; always the reports have been the same.[9] Many who attained that state became the Great Teachers of history and have profoundly influenced human behavior. Such beings, in the course of their comparatively short years, have been capable of creating a realization by millions of people, over millennial periods, of the contextual significance of existence itself. Because these teachings have not concerned the material world as experienced through the senses, they have been labeled "spiritual" or "mystical."[10]

Before the recent interest of scientists in the subject, the study of consciousness was exclusively the concern of spiritual teachers and their students. But in the last twenty years, the considerable interest of numerous theoretical physicists has turned, as we have seen, to the correlation between advanced theoretical physics and the nonmaterial universe. The deepening of popular cultural focus since the 1960s created a receptive audience for spinoffs of this exploration, in such books as Fritjof Capra's *The Tao of Physics*, and Robert Ornstein's *The Psychology of Consciousness*, now classics. The occurrence of higher states of consciousness, traditionally thought to be extremely rare, grows more common as the M-field of the new paradigm spreads; recent surveys indicate that approximately 65 percent of people report having had experiences previously categorized as strictly spiritual.

Because science is by its very nature concerned only with observable phenomena, it has never been attracted to spiritual concepts as a subject for consideration, despite the fact that many great scientists throughout history have personally testified to subjective experiences of pure consciousness occurring in the course of, and frequently crucial to, their work.[11] But the exploding field of nonlinear dynamics provoked curiosity and commentary regarding the nature of existence and consciousness itself, expressed in such books as Ian Stewart's *Does God Play Dice?: The*

Mathematics of Chaos. The new concept of a "science of wholeness" became the subject of popular books such as *Looking Glass Universe*, by John Briggs; and *Turbulent Mirror*, by Briggs and F. David Peat. Recently, astronomers, mathematicians, brain surgeons, and neurologists, as well as physicists, have been caught up in a tide of enthusiasm about the significance of the new discoveries.

We have frequently pointed out that man is unable to observe or recognize an event until there is a prior context and language for naming the event. This inability, called paradigm blindness, is the direct consequence of a limitation of context.[12] Thus it was that the extension of the new intellectual substructure pervading the physical sciences only slowly created the potential for new views and approaches in the "human" sciences, such as psychology.

Although Abraham Maslow long ago discussed "peak experiences," the mainstream literature of psychology never addressed the subject of consciousness itself, with the exception of such classics as *The Varieties of Religious Experience* by William James, which has long been the standard scientific work on the psychology of consciousness as spiritual experience. Eventually, transpersonal psychology went beyond the bounds of experimental and clinical psychology to investigate those aspects of human experience that were purely subjective. Unusual experiences or abilities, once discounted as hoaxes or hallucinations, finally became the subject of parapsychology, legitimizing experimental attempts to verify experiences such as extrasensory perception (ESP).

The field of psychiatry originally arose from the attempt to address the tangible etiology of the intangibles in human behavior and disease. Psychiatry, as a branch of medicine, concerned itself with pathology; therefore, it dealt almost exclusively with the lower levels of consciousness and their neurophysiologic correlates; consciousness as such, however, remained outside the paradigm of classical psychiatry.

In medicine, physicians who worked from a larger paradigm of the healing process and included nontraditional modalities in their therapeutic approaches became known as "holistic" practitioners, a term that at first carried distinct overtones of unprofessionalism among the ranks of the medical establishment. But the contributions of pioneering individuals in this field, especially in such areas as recovery from heart attacks, or the use of prayer to speed up recuperation in surgical patients, demanded serious recognition.

Elisabeth Kübler-Ross brought the attention of the professions, as well as the public, to the phenomena of dying and near-death experiences as reported by patients. Out-of-body experiences also eventually became a relatively common subject, as surgical patients reported out-of-body adventures in which they witnessed their entire operations and heard everything that was said in the operating room.[13] Thelma Moss became well known for her work with Kirlian photography of energy fields, such as those around fingertips. Her photographs of the energy body of a full leaf remaining after it had been cut in two are well known.[14] Eventually, even acupuncture has gained a place of some respect in the American health field, with many physicians learning the technique despite the fact that traditional medicine has not recognized any energies other than mechanical, electrical, or chemical.

Holistic approaches operate from a different context of the nature of human consciousness than does traditional medicine, with emphasis on healing rather than just treating. Though their connection with the theoretical breakthroughs of recent decades may not appear explicit, the alternate therapies employed by holistic health caregivers—whether they are physicians, alternative practitioners, or lay healers, and however widely they differ in their approach and method—all have one common element; all are based on techniques to influence not protoplasm as such, but an *energy field* that surrounds, courses through and influences the human body.[15]

Outside of the medical domain, the phenomenal success of the 12-step self-help movement, to which we have frequently alluded, has impressively established that healing can be effected through the practice of *principles of consciousness*. The capacity to heal desperate conditions, recognized by Carl Jung in his work with Rowland H.—the first link, as we have seen, in the long chain of healings that eventually became the worldwide Alcoholics Anonymous movement—lay distinctly within the realm of higher consciousness. The profound spiritual experience held out as hope by Jung to Rowland, very much akin to the transformations of enlightenment, was the essence of the message passed on to Bill W., the founder of AA.[16] It is notable that Bill W. characterized AA as "the language of the heart."[17]

All these trails, blazed in the pioneering of theoretical and applied human wisdom, have a common point of convergence. Or perhaps it might be better said that they share a common point of origin. Bill W.'s revelation from the depths of despair did not proceed from conceptual rationality or any other introspective focus on self, but rather from a leap to higher consciousness, a transport of Self to the Presence of Infinite Light and Power.[18] That this transformational experience has led to the recovery of millions is merely testimony to the power of energy fields that calibrate at 600 or more. That is the level at which there is a crossover of the experience of consciousness from form to formlessness.

This formless power, the "Higher Power" of the world-wide 12-step self-help movement and the basis for its millions of recoveries,[19] is the same wellspring of power to which all these far-flung branches of intellectual exploration have been not so much thrusting forward, as working their way back. What they are looking for is the power of pure consciousness itself.

CHAPTER 22

Spiritual Struggle

From the understanding of consciousness at which we have arrived, we can reinterpret the struggle of man's spiritual enterprise. Pure consciousness itself, that which is described as "Is-ness," "Being-ness," and "I-am-ness," represents the infinite potential, infinite power, and infinite energy source of all existence, identified as "Deity," "God," "Divinity." Within this potential, the Unmanifest becomes Manifest as the Avatar—the Christ, the Buddha, the Great Teacher, the Great Guru— whose energy field calibrates at 1,000. These individuals set up attractor patterns of enormous power to which the mind, with its holographic capacity to react globally to attractor fields, is subject.

Of lesser moment but still enormously powerful, are the enlightened teachers who have taught the path to the realization of the "Self." The Self has been described by the enlightened throughout time as infinite, formless, changeless, all-present, unmanifest-and-manifest.[1] Herein is the Oneness, the Allness, and Godness of all that exists, indistinguishable from the Creator, whose power in the human realm is a giant attractor field that allows and encompasses variation (free will) so that, in the end, "all paths lead to Me." Teachings and other works that treat of this typically calibrated at 700 in our studies.

At the energy field of 600, ordinary thought ceases. Beyond temporal linear process, existence is witnessed as Knowingness, omnipresence, and nonduality. Because existence itself has no locality, the "me/you" duality and consequent illusion of separation disappear.[2] This state is the peace beyond all understanding, infinite, unconditional love—all-encompassing, all-knowing, all-present, omni-powerful, and concordant with the Self, which is the awareness that the Manifest is one with the Unmanifest.

Truly spiritual states can be said to begin at a calibrated level of about 500 (Love), become Unconditional Love at 540, and then continue on to infinity. Teachers who calibrate in the high 500s and the 600s are frequently recognized as saints; their state of consciousness is often described as sublime.[3]

It is a not uncommon experience for students to enter into such a sublime state when in the presence of teachers whose energy fields calibrate at 550 and over, through the process of "entrainment," which is the dominance of a powerful attractor field. Until the devotee arrives at the higher state of awareness, this state will not persist when not in the higher energy field of the teacher.[4] Advanced spiritual seekers often fluctuate in and out of this "presence of the Beloved" as they approach enlightenment; this loss of the higher state and descent to a lower is identified in both Eastern and Western literature as an "anguish of the soul."[5]

Spiritual work, like other intensive pursuits, can be arduous and frequently requires the development of specific tools for the task, including an extremely focused intent and unfailing concentration. The difficulty of inner work results from the great effort required to escape from the familiar gravity of lower attractor fields and move to the influence of a higher field. In order to ameliorate this struggle, all religions issue proscriptions against exposing oneself to the lower energy fields; it is only from an authoritarian viewpoint that such error is depicted as "sin." A more liberal viewpoint accepts man's dalliance in lower energy fields as pardonable "failings." But attitudes emotions, and behaviors characteristic of the energy fields below 200 do, in fact, generally preclude spiritual experience.

The classical chakra system recognized by many spiritual disciplines correlates almost exactly with the Map of Consciousness that has emerged from our studies. The level of 600 corresponds to the crown chakra, level 525 to the third eye chakra, level 505 to the heart chakra, level 350 to the throat chakra, level 275 to the solar plexus and the spleen or sacral chakras, and level 200 to the base or root chakra (calibrations in 2010).

All spiritual teachings advise against "worldliness," suggesting avoidance of attachment to sex or money, as well as avoidance of lower attitudes and emotions such as spite, envy, resentment, and jealousy. Absorption with such lower fields prohibits spiritual progress.[6]

The lower regions are also the locus of addictions; one can be fixated at any of the lower levels. Almost all of these energy fields, and the behaviors associated with them, now have given rise to specific self-help groups, all of which concur that without a spiritual context, recovery is quite unlikely, if not impossible. In consciousness-raising programs in general, a universal dictum is that one is powerless until one tells the truth. All spiritually oriented self-help groups require this first step. They are unanimous that an open mind and willingness are necessary prerequisites to progress; in other words, one must have reached an energy field of 200 in one's own inner development to be healable. Lingering within the influence of fields below this entails a real danger of becoming so deeply entrained that one cannot escape. This is not always so, however; history has noted many occasions of individuals in the very depths of such entrainment who suddenly break through to a high level of consciousness.

Such sudden breakthroughs are still seen on occasion in modern society; this, as we have seen, was the precise experience of Bill W., which resulted in the founding of AA. This experience seems typically to be characterized by a total transformation of consciousness, liberation from the entrainment of lower attractor fields and a sudden emergence into higher awareness. (This type of experience, common in the early days of AA, when its members were frequently "last-gaspers," is not reported by "high bottom" members, who constitute the majority of newcomers to AA today.)

Just as the entrainment or influence of the higher energy fields has an anabolic, or growth-enhancing, effect on a subject, entrainment by lower attractor fields has the opposite, a catabolic or destructive effect; the most widespread example in today's culture is the influence of some forms of violent rap music. Among our test subjects, punk rock, death rock, and gangster rap music made every subject go weak, confirming earlier observations made by Dr. John Diamond.[7] In a more recent study of students (reported in *The Arizona Republic*, July 4, 1994), Dr. James Johnson of the University of North Carolina found that rap music increases tolerance for and predisposition to violence, while promoting materialism and reducing both immediate interest in academics, and long-term success.

A common experience observed in therapy groups and clinics is that drug abusers do not recover if they continue to listen to heavy metal rock music; a one-year follow-up of inpatient and outpatient cocaine addicts from Sedona Villa, a branch of Camelback Hospital of Phoenix, Arizona, indicated that not a single cocaine abuser who continued to listen to this kind of violent and negative music recovered.[8] Self-help groups for the addicted invariably recommend avoiding the influence (that is, the energy fields) of former lifestyle associates. These addicts found that just leaving the drug was not enough; to do so was merely to attack the A→B→C of addiction. As long as they could not make the commitment of will to entirely leave the influence of the field—of which the music, like the drug, was simply a manifestation—they could not escape entrainment to the low-energy attractor, the ABC of addiction.

Recovered addicts who leave the energy field of their self-help programs rather predictably relapse.[9] Besides having relinquished the infusion of the combined power of their fellow members, their assertion that they can "go it alone" is a notorious symptom of an oncoming relapse as the ego arises, because it indicates an infiltration of arrogance and pride, calibrating at 175, which is below the power of the energy field required for healing.

The same principle, of course, operates in the other direction. To seek enlightenment is to seek entrainment to the most powerful attractor patterns. The key, again, is will, a constantly repeated act of choice. Here, the chaos-theory principle of sensitive dependence on initial conditions provides a scientific explanation of the traditional way of spiritual progress. In all spiritual disciplines, the opening wedge predicated for advancing one's awareness is described as "willingness." History shows what has been clinically known as well: persistent willingness is the trigger that activates a new attractor field and allows one to begin to leave the old. We may visualize a lesser attractor field approaching a greater one, at which point the introduction of a third element (such as free will) suddenly creates a crossover (a "saddle-pattern"), and the change takes place.

In Eastern spiritual disciplines, it is accepted that the devotee alone, unaided by a guru or a teacher, is unlikely to make much progress.[10] The AA experience is that a true alcoholic is unable to recover without the help of a sponsor. In sports, great coaches are sought after because their influence inspires maximum effort. A devotee can abet his own progress by merely focusing on an advanced teacher and thereby aligning with that teacher's energy field; in our testing, it was shown repeatedly that holding in mind the image of an advanced spiritual teacher made every subject go strong, irrespective of their personal beliefs.

The agency of change in spiritual struggles of personal metamorphosis is always beyond the power of the seeker. Great saints, such as Francis of Assisi, have

typically asserted that they were mere channels of a
higher power from without, and took no credit for
personal initiative or achievement of their own state,
which they attributed solely to Grace.[11] This is illustra-
tive of the instrumentation whereby the newcomer
from a lesser level of awareness, who places himself in
the influence of a higher awareness, is transformed "by
osmosis" (entrainment). Even casual observers frequently note this conspicuous absence of agency on
the part of the person so clearly transmuted by an
invisible force.

When someone suddenly goes from the influence
of a lower attractor field to that of a higher, it is often
acclaimed as a miracle. The unfortunate verdict of
human experience is that few escape the energy fields
that gradually come to dominate their behaviors. A
currently popular spiritual program designed to
facilitate such escape is "A Course in Miracles."[12] The
purpose of this course of spiritual psychology is to
prepare the necessary groundwork to precipitate a
sudden jump in consciousness through encouraging
a total change of perception. In more traditional fashion, prayer and meditation also provide points of
departure to rise from the influence of a lower energy
field into a higher.

Physicians who themselves calibrate at 500 and
over become powerful healers, and they accomplish
striking successes with treatments with which others
are unable to achieve similar results (and thereby producing paradoxical data in many so-called double-blind
studies). Such inexplicable variances show the intervention of power unaccountable by the routine, causal

explanation that predominates in medical science. In a holographic world, any "single" event is actually the result of all events in the universe; "events" as such have no self-existent reality. The universe *is* man's consciousness. It requires a comprehension beyond that of just the intellect alone.

The achievements of pure reason are the great landmarks of cultural history. They have made man the master of his external environment, and to some degree, on the physical plane, of his internal environment. But reason has its limits, in more ways than one. The intellectual brilliance of the 400 level, so dazzling and enviable to those in the 300s, quickly palls for those who have transcended it. From a higher perspective, it is all too clear how tedious and trivial reason's infatuation with itself can become. Reason is the mirror of the mind's vanity; ultimately, there are few things more boring to observe than self-admiration.

Rationality, the great liberator that has freed us from the demands of our lower natures, is also a stern warden, denying our escape to the planes above and beyond intellect. For those entrained at the level of the 400s, reason itself becomes the cap, a ceiling in spiritual evolution. It is striking how many of history's great names calibrate at 499—Descartes, Newton, Einstein, and dozens more. It is a final sticking point, an enormous barrier; the fight to overcome it is the most common, and frequently the lengthiest, of spiritual struggles.

It is not unheard of for very advanced scientists, thoroughly entrained by the influences of the level of Reason, to have sudden breakthroughs and emerge into a realm of global awareness and wholeness.[13] The world of spirituality is coincident with the world of nondeterministic science and nonlinear systems, as we have attempted to show. Our research and this presentation, in fact, are designed to facilitate rational recognition of spiritual phenomena by those who are predominantly linear and habituated to the "left-brain" modality. Perhaps the construct of our map of the anatomy of consciousness can illuminate somewhat the nature of ultimate causality by illustrating that the power of creation proceeds from the top down, rather than from the bottom up.

It is our hope, though, not to dogmatize, but to assist the reader in a process of self-revelation, as it is our desire to address not merely that figment designated as the reader's rational self, but his entire consciousness. In our study, it is the total person that reacts to the test stimuli. Although the subject's mind may not be aware of what is going on, his total being certainly is, or there would be no consistency to our findings. This reminds us of the observation of advanced spiritual teachers, that the devotee has only to discover...that which he already knows.

CHAPTER 23

The Search for Truth

Cynical though it may at first sound, we must admit that for everyday operational purposes, truth is whatever is subjectively convincing at one's current level of perception. At the lower levels of consciousness, propositions are accepted as true even when they are illogical, unfounded, and express tenets neither intellectually provable nor practically demonstrable. This is not a phenomenon restricted to the "lunatic fringe." Far more often than we would like to admit, innocent persons are convicted and jailed on the testimony of clearly irrational or biased witnesses. Globally, the basis for perennial wars (such as those in Slavic Europe or the Middle East) is an insane belief in the justice of revenge, which virtually guarantees endless conflict.

With few exceptions, even religions that ostensibly represent the teachings of the "Prince of Peace" have never forbidden war or the killing of other human beings under "justifiable" circumstances—justifiable, of course, to those doing the killing; their victims would likely fail to appreciate the justification. Such self-contradictory behavior, diametrically opposed to the underlying principles of a faith, will appear less surprising if we apply critical factor analysis to calibrate the evolution, or devolution, of spiritual teachings over time.

We can look at the world's foremost religious teachings in this way.

(Note on calibration differences: The calibrations of religious groups change over time consequent to changes in their policies. In this revised edition, therefore, we include calibrations from the 2005 book *Truth vs. Falsehood* in parentheses. *Truth vs. Falsehood* was published ten years after *Power vs. Force* and provides extended discussions and calibrations of particular religious groups, spiritual practices, and scriptural writings. Also, when a subject is calibrated multiple times, this re-addressing may contribute to a change in calibration.)

Christianity
The level of truth originally expounded by Jesus Christ calibrates at 1,000, the highest attainable on this plane. By the second century though, the level of truth of the practice of his teachings had dropped to 930, and by the sixth century, had dropped to 540. By the time of the crusades, at the beginning of the eleventh century, it had fallen to its current level of 498. A major decline in the year 325 A.D. was apparently due to the spread of misinterpretations of the teachings originating from the Council of Nicaea. Students of religious history will find it interesting to calibrate the level of truth of Christianity as practiced before and after Paul, Constantine, Augustine, etc.[1]

It should be noted that the Lamsa translation, from the Aramaic, of the New Testament calibrates at 750, whereas the King James version, from the Greek, is 500. Just as there is a wide range in the level of truth of various translations, so there is a wide variation between different Christian practices. Most major persuasions—Roman Catholicism, Anglicanism, Christian Science and many small denominations, such as the Quakers—calibrate in the high 500s. (In 2005, calibrations of the principal Christian denominations ranged from 310 to 535.) Specialized interpretations, such as that of the contemporary *A Course in Miracles* on the one hand, or the 14th-century mysticism of Meister Eckhart on the other hand, calibrate at 600-700. As in the case of Islam, however, extreme fundamentalist groups with explicit reactionary political agendas can calibrate as low as 125, or even much lower.

Buddhism
The level of truth of the teachings of the Buddha was also originally at 1,000. By the sixth century A.D., the level of truth in practice, however, had dropped to an average of 900. These teachings have deteriorated less than any other religion: Hinayana Buddhism (the lesser vehicle) still calibrates at 850; Mahayana Buddhism (the greater vehicle) calibrates at 950; current practice of Zen Buddhism is in the 600s. (In 2005, calibrations of the principal branches within Buddhism ranged from 405 to 960.)

Hinduism
The teachings of Lord Krishna calibrated at 1,000 and have deteriorated very slowly over time, so that the truth of the current practice still calibrates at 850 or over.   (In 2005, calibrations of the principal Yogas ranged from "Hatha Yoga" at 390 to "Jnana Yoga" at 975.)

Judaism
The teachings of Abraham calibrated at 985; the practice current at the time of Moses calibrated at 770; the

level of truth of the Talmud calibrates at 665 (calibrated 2011). Modern Judaism calibrates at 499. (In 2005, calibrations of the principal branches within Judaism ranged from 550 to 605, with the Zohar calibrating at 905.). The Old Testament calibrates at about 475.

Islam

The level of consciousness of Mohammed varied. The Koran calibrates at 700 (calibrated 2011). The kernel of Islamic faith is an expression of loving acceptance and inner peace, but the evolution of practical dogma was intertwined from the start with the politics of territorial expansion in the form of *jihad*, or religious warfare. The truth of the teachings had dropped severely by the end of the Crusades. In modern times, the ascendance of fanatic nationalistic religious movements, characterized by paranoia and xenophobia, has rapidly eroded the spiritual essence of this faith. At the present time, the level of truth of the teachings of militant Islamic fundamentalism varies between 90 to 130. (In 2005, calibrations of Islam ranged from Wahhabism at 30 to Sufism at 700.)

———•———

When we look at the decline of the level of truth of the world's great religions, we notice that those which are the most "yin" have remained relatively pure throughout the ages, whereas those which are more "yang" (involved in worldly affairs) have degraded markedly, until the militant extremist faction of the most aggressive religions has actually sunk below the critical level of integrity at 200. The more dualistic the creed, the

greater seems to be its vulnerability to misinterpretation. Dualism promotes a split between belief and
action, and the discernment of levels of truth. When
this occurs, the spiritual essence can be confused in
translation into physical expression. Thus, the conceptual Christian Soldier (of the spirit) becomes, through a
distorted "literal" translation, a self-justified battlefield
killer.

The Hindus did not fall into the error of confusing
levels of interpretation; the battle described in the
opening of the *Bhagavad Gita* was never misinterpreted to suggest Lord Krishna teaches that believers are to
engage in actual warfare. The Buddha's view—that the
cause of all pain and suffering is ignorance, which he
saw as the only "sin" possible, and that one's duty is to
be compassionate toward others and pray for them—is
hardly susceptible to such distortion.

The downfall of all lofty spiritual teachings has
been their misinterpretation by the less enlightened;
each level of consciousness predefines its own limited
capacity for perception and comprehension. Until one
has oneself become enlightened, or at least experienced the higher states of consciousness, all spiritual
teachings remain hearsay and are thus prone to distortion and misunderstanding. Scripture can be quoted to
justify any position. The "righteous" are always dangerous because of their imbalanced perception and their
consequent indifference to moral violence. Within any
religion, fundamentalist sects always calibrate lowest,
often operating at the same level of consciousness as
criminality; their hallmark is egocentric extremism and
irrationality. But with 85 percent of the human popula-

tion calibrating below the critical level of 200, error is easily disseminated and readily accepted around the world.

Cults proliferate because the general public has no objective criteria with which to distinguish truth from falsehood. Using the tools of this study, we may identify as a "cult" any purportedly spiritual movement that calibrates below the level of 200. As we have seen above, cults are not just isolated, renegade phenomena; they also thrive as tolerated subgroups within the world's great religions, distorting teachings and subverting their intent.

Cults indeed need not be formally religious at all. The ultimate cult, of course, is that of anti-religion based on anti-divinity, known as "Satanism." It has no explicit religious agenda of its own, as it defines itself through antithesis and reversal of benign principles. In one form or another, it has always been with us. As up implies down and light implies darkness, man's socially organized search for truth and commitment to higher spiritual levels has always implied the socially organized promulgation of falsehood and submission to the lowest energy fields. Examination of the nature of anti-religion demonstrates, in fact, the enormously destructive power of negative energy fields. Examples are unfortunately ready at hand.

The trappings of disguised Satanism spread as fashions of a popular youth subculture, its primary vehicle being an overt musical style. But principles are implicit in trappings, and principles generate attractor fields. The effects are all too familiar to any clinician practicing near an urban area. The destruction of energy fields is pathogenic. Victims become desensitized to distinctions between good and evil, a value inversion that can be clinically examined. Habitués are found to directly display "blown-out" acupuncture systems and desynchronization of the cerebral hemispheres in response to repetitive negative patterns of the associated music. The net result is, in effect, a hypnotic trance during which the listener is highly susceptible to the violent and blasphemous suggestion of the lyrics. In this sense, these children become literally enslaved, prone to later bouts of irrational destruction in which they, in truth, "don't know why" they act as they do, as they are acting out unconscious, post-hypnotic suggestions. But the influence persists.

Continued weakening of the body and its immune system long after the music stops is accompanied by an inversion of kinesiologic response. Negative stimuli that would make a normal person go weak paradoxically cause a strong response, while those that would make a normal person go strong now produce a weak one. Unaware that they are the victims of a potent negative energy field, the members of this subculture sink into sometimes inescapable subservience to forces beyond their comprehension. Youth subjected to such physical, emotional, and sexual abuse can suffer permanent damage to the brain's neurotransmitter balance, becoming adult depressives who habitually seek out abusive partners and must endlessly struggle against an inclination to suicide that is, in fact, a lingering form of post-hypnotic suggestion.[2]

We may wish to deny that such a spiritual plague, reminiscent of the Dark Ages, could still remain virulent

in our seemingly enlightened society. But such perverse influences do not operate in a moral vacuum or
arise from a social matrix that does not already incorporate preconditions for their growth. The paradox of
a puritanical society is that it encourages constant
seduction but denies satisfaction, so a perpetual frustration of normal outlets eventually finds release in perverse ones. If we look more closely, we may find that
other elements of what we call "civilization" in fact also
foster its persistence.

———

While the young are being programmed by the specialized TV and computer games that glorify violence, their
parents are being brainwashed by adult media.
Kinesiologic testing showed that a fairly typical TV
show caused test subjects to go weak multiple times
during a single episode. Each of these weakening
events suppressed the observer's immune system. Each
weakening reflected an insult to the viewer's central as
well as autonomic nervous systems. Invariably accompanying each of these disruptions of the acupuncture
system were suppressions of the thymus gland; each
insult also resulted in damage to the brain's delicate
neurohormonal and neurotransmitter systems. Each
negative input brought the watcher closer to eventual
sickness and to depression—now one of the world's
most prevalent illnesses.

Subtle grades of subclinical depression kill more
people than all the other illnesses of mankind combined. There is no antidepressant that will cure a
depression that is spiritually based, because the malaise

does not originate from brain dysfunction, but from an accurate response to the desecration of life. The body is the reflection of the spirit in its physical expression, and its problems are dramatization of the struggles of the spirit that gives it life. A belief that we ascribe to "out there" has its effect "in here." Everyone dies by his own hand. That is a hard clinical fact, not a moral view.

———

The attempt to impose standards of would-be absolute Good and Evil is, in fact, one of the great moral pitfalls. But without moralizing, we can plainly state that whatever calibrates above 200 supports life and may therefore be functionally defined as "good;" whereas, whatever calibrates below 200 is destructive, non-supportive of life and can thus be declared functionally "negative." By testing, we can prove that a false premise such as "the end justifies the means" is operationally negative, yet this is a routinely accepted justification for much of human behavior, from the peccadilloes of commerce to the enormities of war. Such spiritual ambiguity, leading ultimately to irretrievable confusion between functional good and evil, has always been the Achilles' heel of human society.

It is this process of perversion of truth through a failure of discernment that has provided the instrumentation of the decline in the world's great religions (as noted above). Religions that fall below the level of 500 may preach love, but they will not be able to practice it. And no religious system that encourages war can claim spiritual authority without the blatant hypocrisy that has made atheists of many honest men.

Society is collectively most vulnerable when the capacity to distinguish between attractors and imitators, or to perceive nuances of differing levels of consciousness, is dulled. This is how civil abuses become law and political extremists persuade with righteous slogans. The children of violence become its perpetrators because a confused society that has lost the capacity for discernment necessary to protect its own consciousness can hardly hope to protect its young.

An individual's level of consciousness is determined by the principles to which they are committed. To maintain progress in consciousness, there can be no wavering about principle, or the individual will fall back to a lower level. Expediency is never an adequate justification. If it is wrong to kill another human being, that principle can allow no exceptions, regardless of how emotionally appealing a construct may be used to justify the exception. Thus, a society that condones capital punishment will always have a problem with murder. Both are products of the same level of perception. To the murderer, the killing of the victim is also a justifiable exception.

Once a principle is breached, its mutated form propagates like cancer. A society that supports killing, whether in war, or by the police, or by the penal system, cannot at the same time effectively stop "criminal" killing. To kill is to kill is to kill; there is no escaping that fact. The decision to kill or not is a basic issue on the path to real power; but this rudimentary step has not even been essayed by 85 percent of the world's population or by virtually any of its governments. Koko, the famous gorilla who was a resident of the

Primate Research Institute, has worked for some years with a psychologist and developed a sophisticated sign language vocabulary. She is truthful, affectionate, intelligent, and trustworthy; her integrity calibrates at 250. Thus, one is safer with Koko, a gorilla, than with 85 percent of the humans on the planet.

Injury to man's "spiritual eye" has resulted in dimness of moral vision and blindness to truth, which afflicts 85 percent of the earth's population who linger below the critical level of integrity. The great issue that confronts mankind as a whole is the healing of this spiritual blindness. The more immediate "problem" of so-called Right and Wrong that always diverts our societal focus only exists as a function of perception based at the lower levels of consciousness. Little children are taught that dangerous behaviors are "wrong," but as they grow older, discernment should replace moralism. Whether or not it is wrong to kill other human beings may be a moral dilemma at lower levels of consciousness; at higher levels the very question is ridiculous and not even conceivable. Conventional morality is, therefore, only a provisional substitute for a faculty of higher consciousness. Moralism, a by-product of duality, becomes insignificant as the consciousness level rises through the 500s, and becomes irrelevant at the level of 600.

Merely to reach a stage where one functions primarily from reason requires a major evolution in consciousness to the 400s, which is a very powerful level in world society. Freud, Einstein, and Descartes calibrated at 499, which is also the level of humanism.[3] But reason, so vulnerable to loss of perspective through self-absorption, has in the long run never provided man with any solid moral, or even intellectual, certitude. Again and again it has, to the contrary, led from the chaos of ignorance to an equally baffling cerebral maze. In a world of mass confusion, we desperately need a reliable, accurate, objectively verifiable yardstick with which to measure truth. Hopefully, this study has presented such a tool. Any increased infusion of the influence of truth into the collective human consciousness gives us cause for greater hope than may be apparent from what tends inevitably to be a rather gloomy overview.

We have established that consciousness is capable of discerning any change of energy to a degree of log 10 (to the minus infinity). This means that there is no possible event in the entire universe that is not detectable by the exquisite sensitivity of consciousness itself. The energy of human thought, though minute, is nonetheless absolutely measurable. A thought that emanates from the consciousness level 100 will typically measure between log $10^{-800 \text{ million}}$ to $10^{-700 \text{ million}}$ microwatts. On the other hand, a loving thought at the consciousness level of 500 measures approximately log $10^{-35 \text{ million}}$ microwatts.

Although only 15 percent of the world's population is above the critical consciousness level of 200, the collective power of that 15 percent has the weight to counterbalance the negativity of the remaining 85 percent of the world's population. Because the scale of power advances logarithmically, a single Avatar at a consciousness level of 1,000 can and does, in fact, totally counterbalance the collective negativity of all of mankind. Kinesiologic testing has shown that:

One individual at level 700	counterbalances	70 million individuals below level 200
One individual at level 600	counterbalances	10 million individuals below level 200
One individual at level 500	counterbalances	750,000 individuals below level 200
One individual at level 400	counterbalances	400,000 individuals below level 200
One individual at level 300	counterbalances	90,000 individuals below level 200
12 individuals at level 700	equals	one Avatar at 1,000

At the original writing of this book, there were twelve persons on the planet who calibrated over 600. In May, 2006, however, there were only six: three between 600-700, one between 700-800, one between 800-900, and one between 900-1,000.

Were it not for these counterbalances, mankind would self-destruct out of the sheer mass of its unopposed negativity. However, the difference in power between a loving thought ($10^{-35 \text{ million}}$ microwatts) and a fearful thought ($10^{-750 \text{ million}}$ microwatts) is so enormous as to be beyond the capacity of the human imagination to even comprehend. We can see from the analysis

above that even a few loving thoughts during the
course of the day more than counterbalance all of our
negative thoughts by their sheer power.

From a social-behavioral viewpoint, as we said,
truth is a set of principles by which people live, regardless of what they might say they believe. We have seen
that there is subjective truth, operational truth, hypo-
thetical truth, and intellectual truth; and then there is
factual truth. The legitimacy of any of these is
dependent on the context of a given perceptual level.
Truth is not functional unless it is meaningful, and
meaning, like value, is dependent on a unique perceptual field. Facts and data may be convincing at one
level and irrelevant at another. Functional validity of
information received also varies with the intellectual
level and capacity for abstraction of the mind of the
recipient. To be operational, truth must not simply be
"true" but knowable; yet each level of truth is unknowable to the levels below it and has no validity beyond
its own territory. Thus, we can conclude that all
kinds of truth as we know it within the dimension of
ordinary human function are examples of *dependent
truth*, whose veracity is totally contingent on a given
set of parameters, or context. Even our revered "scientific truth" is also truth by definition only under certain
conditions, and therefore subject to dispute and error.
Statistical inference has become a propaganda tool,
and the statistical distortions by which anything can
be proven about anything have alienated our credence.

Is there any impersonal truth, independent of
individual condition or context?

Truth, as detected by the research methods

explained throughout this book, derives its validity from ultimate sources far beyond the influence of any localized perceptual field. It represents neither personality nor opinion and does not vary with any condition of test subject or environment.

Ignorance does not yield to attack, but it dissipates in the light, and nothing dissolves dishonesty faster than the simple act of revealing the truth. The only way to enhance one's power in the world is by increasing one's integrity, understanding, and capacity for compassion. If the diverse populations of mankind can be brought to this realization, the survival of human society and the happiness of its members are more secure.

The initial effect of taking responsibility for the truth of one's life is to raise lower energy field levels to 200, the critical level at which power first appears, and the stepping-stone to all of the higher levels. The Courage to face truth leads eventually to Acceptance, where greater power arises at the level of 350. Here, then, there is sufficient energy to solve the majority of man's social problems. This, in turn, leads to the yet greater power available at 500, the level of Love. Knowing our own and everyone else's human foibles gives rise to forgiveness, and thence to compassion. Compassion is the doorway to Grace, to the final realization of who we are and why we are here, and the ultimate source of all existence.

CHAPTER 24

Resolution

A thorough absorption of the material presented here-in has been shown to be able to raise one's level of consciousness by an average of 35 points. Inasmuch as the progression of consciousness during the average human lifetime lived on this planet has been only 5 points, such an increase of 35 in individual awareness is of enormous benefit in and of itself. And, as advanced theoretical physics and nonlinear dynamics have shown, any individual increase also raises to some degree the consciousness of everyone on the planet.

To become more conscious is the greatest gift anyone can give to the world; moreover, in a ripple effect, the gift comes back to its source. While the level of consciousness of mankind as a whole stood at a perilous 190 for many centuries, in the mid-1980s, it suddenly jumped to the hopeful level of 204. For the first time in history, man is now on safe ground from which to continue his upward march. And this promise of new hope comes none too soon.

Today, many of the subjects we have discussed are exploding in the news media. The perversion of religion to the ends of political savagery, the deepening depravity of crimes, the involvement of children in violence, moral confusion in politics, and the bizarre violence of cults all appear against a backdrop colored by the prevalence of lies as social tender, and a lack of consensus as to individual and collective responsibility towards one's fellow man.

This social confusion and paralysis stems from the dearth of guidelines upon which to base decisions.

307

Hopefully, this book has taken a step toward filling that void with what is, in fact, an essay on the science of Morality. By "Morality," we do not refer to merely petty moralistic judgments of right and wrong, but to an at once objective and personal basis from which to make decisions and evaluations regarding the highest conduct of our lives.

In a social framework, we can certainly choose to refuse passive acquiescence to any political system that falls below the level of 200. Instead, applying our newly developed faculties of examination and correction, it is now possible, for instance, to establish clear criteria by which holders of public office should be selected. Each office requires a specific minimum level of awareness in order to be effective; in general, any government official who falls below 200 will not solve problems but create them.

The larger social issue is how, in view of the dark side of mankind's behavior, one can maintain compassion. It is a relative world; everyone acts from his own level of truth and therefore believes that his own actions and decisions are "right"; it is this very "rightness" that makes fanatics so dangerous. But the real danger to society does not come from overt bigotry such as white supremacism (which calibrates at 150), as such damage can at least be monitored. The really grave danger to society lies in the silent and invisible entrainment that stealthily conquers the psyche. In the process of entrainment of the public consciousness, negative attractor fields are cosmeticized by rhetoric and the manipulation of symbols. Moreover, it is not the overt message of the negative input that destroys consciousness, but the energy field that accompanies it.

The extreme negativity of many popular works of pseudo-philosophy, for example, is obvious if one tests these books. But even being forewarned cannot defend us against unwitting entrainment by invisible energy fields that are activated when these works are read. One may think that he can maintain his psychic independence by refuting the work intellectually, but mere exposure to the material has a profound negative effect that continues even after the material is intellectually rejected. It is as though there is within these negative influences a hidden virus whose invasion of our psyche goes unnoticed and undetected.

Additionally, we often relax our circumspection when encountering material that ascribes to itself the attributes of spiritual insight or religion, forgetting that every heinous crime of which man is capable has been perpetrated in the name of God. While violent cults may be clearly repellent, belief systems that masquerade as piety are even more insidious, for they corrupt by the silent entrainment of invisible attractor fields.

Here, it is best to heed the traditional wisdom that tells us not to fear evil or fight it, but merely to avoid it; yet in order to avoid it, one has to have the capacity to recognize it. Socrates said, in effect, that without such capacity, youth (including the youth that continues to reside within every adult) is corrupted by low-energy attractor fields. Although Socrates was put to death for teaching this discernment, his teaching remains: obscurity is dispelled by augmenting the light of discernment, not by attacking the darkness.[1] The final issue, then, is the problem of how we may best cultivate and preserve the power of moral discernment.

Our journey of investigation has finally led us to the most critical realization of all: *Mankind lacks the capacity to recognize the difference between good and evil.*

By humbly surrendering to this awareness, man may be forearmed. When we admit that we are gullible and easily seduced by the senses and deluded by glamour (including intellectual glamour), we have at least the beginning of discernment. Fortunately, in this world of duality, man has been given a consciousness that can instantly detect that which is destructive, and signal it to his otherwise ignorant mind by the grossly visible weakening of his body in the presence of inimical stimuli. Wisdom can ultimately be reduced to the simple process of avoiding that which makes you go weak—nothing else is really required.

Through frequent practice of this technique, spiritual blindness to the discernment of truth and falsehood can be progressively replaced by a growing intuitive vision. Some lucky few seem born with this innate capacity; their lives remain clear and undamaged by negative entrainment. But for most of us, life has not been that easy; we have spent a great deal of time repairing the damage done by destructive attractor fields that have acted almost unconsciously and hypnotically. Recovering even from a single addiction can take up the majority of a single lifetime—and the most common and insidious addiction is to denial, which plagues all of mankind through intellectual vanity.

The intellect, contrary to its delusions of grandeur, not only lacks the ability to recognize falsehood, but lacks the necessary power to defend itself, even if it had the capacity of discernment. Is it irreverent, in light of history's enormous accretion of works of intellectual speculation, to say that man's vaunted capacity of reason lacks that critical faculty of discernment? The whole field of philosophy is merely evidence that man has struggled and failed for thousands of years to arrive at the simplest recognition of what is true and what is false, or the discourse would long ago have reached some consensus.

And it is clear from common human conduct that even if the intellect could reliably arrive at this basic conclusion, *it still lacks the power to stop the effect of negative fields*. We remain unconscious of the causes of our afflictions while the intellect dreams up all kinds of plausible excuses, hypnotized itself by these same forces. Even when a person intellectually knows his behavior is self-destructive, this knowledge has no necessary deterrent effect whatsoever; intellectual recognition of our addictions has never given us the power to control them.

In scripture, we are told that man is afflicted by forces unseen.[2] It is a commonplace observation of our century that silent, invisible rays of energy are emitted even by innocent-looking objects; the discoverers of radium paid for this realization with their lives. X-rays are lethal, and radioactive emissions kill silently, as does radon. The attractor energy fields that destroy us are equally invisible and no less powerful, though far more subtle.

When it is said that someone is "possessed," what is meant is that his consciousness has become dominated

by negative attractor fields from which the person cannot extricate himself. By this definition, we can see
that whole segments of society are so thoroughly
"possessed" that they themselves are unconscious of
their motives. Wisdom tells us that one worships either
heaven or hell and will eventually become the servant
of one or the other. Hell is not a condition imposed by
a judgmental God, but rather the inevitable consequence of one's own decisions. Hell is the final outcome of constantly choosing the negative and thus
isolating oneself from love and truth.

Enlightened beings have always described the
general populace as being "trapped in a dream"; the
majority of people are driven by unseen forces, and
most are in despair over this fact for a great deal of
their lives. We pray to God to relieve us of the burden
of our sins, and by confession, we look for relief.
Remorse seems woven into the fabric of life. How
can salvation be possible, then, for those who have
unwittingly become ensnared in such destructive
influences?

In fact, however, even from a merely scientific viewpoint, salvation is indeed possible; in truth, it is guaran-
teed by the simple fact that the energy of a loving
thought is enormously more powerful than that of a
negative one. Therefore, the traditional solutions of
love and prayer have a sound scientific basis; man has
within his own essence the power of his own salvation.

Humanity could be called an affliction with which
we are all burdened. We do not remember asking to
be born, and we inherited a mind so limited that it is
hardly capable of distinguishing between that which

embraces life and that which leads to death.[3] The whole struggle of life is in transcending this myopia. We cannot enter into higher levels of existence until we advance in consciousness to the point where we overcome duality and are no longer earthbound. Perhaps it is because of our collective will to transcend that we have earned the capacity to finally discover an inborn compass to lead us out of the darkness of ignorance. We needed something very simple, which could bypass those traps of the wily intellect for which we have paid such an enormous price. This compass merely says "yes" or "no." It tells us that what is aligned with heaven makes us go strong and what is aligned with hell makes us go weak.

The ubiquitous human ego is actually not an "I" at all; it is merely an "it." Seeing through this illusion reveals an endless Cosmic Joke, in which the human tragedy itself is part of the comedy. The irony of human experience is in how fiercely the ego fights to preserve the illusion of being a separate, individual "I," even though this is not only an ontological impossibility, but the very wellspring of all suffering. Human reason exhausts itself ceaselessly to explain the inexplicable. Explanation itself is high comedy, as preposterous as trying to see the back of one's own head, but the vanity of the ego is boundless, and it becomes even more overblown in this very attempt to make sense of nonsense. The mind, in its identity with the ego, cannot, by definition, comprehend reality; if it could, it would instantly dissolve itself upon recognition of its own illusory nature and basis. It is only beyond the paradox of mind transcending ego that what Is stands forth as self-evident and dazzling in its infinite Absoluteness. And then all of these words are useless.

But perhaps from compassion for each other's blindness, we can learn to forgive ourselves, and peace can then be our assured future. Our purpose on Earth may remain obscure, but the road henceforth is clear. With the consciousness level of humanity now finally above 200, we may expect great transformations throughout human culture, as mankind becomes more responsible for its knowledge, and thus its deeds. We have become fully accountable, whether we like it or not. We are at the point in the evolution of our collective awareness where we may even assume stewardship of consciousness itself. Humanity is no longer resigned to passively paying the price of ignorance, or its communal consciousness would not have risen to its new level. From this time forth, man may choose to no longer be enslaved by darkness; his destiny can then be certain.

Gloria in Excelsis Deo!

Appendices

APPENDIX A

CALIBRATION OF THE TRUTH OF THE CHAPTERS

Overall Calibration of Book: 850

Chapter 1 780		Chapter 13 870	
Chapter 2 830		Chapter 14 870	
Chapter 3 750		Chapter 15 730	
Chapter 4 770		Chapter 16 760	
Chapter 5 740		Chapter 17 770	
Chapter 6 710		Chapter 19 830	
Chapter 7 740		Chapter 18 770	
Chapter 8 820		Chapter 20 890	
Chapter 9 800		Chapter 21 870	
Chapter 10 780		Chapter 22 860	
Chapter 11 770		Chapter 23 880	
Chapter 12 800		Chapter 24 860	

MAP OF CONSCIOUSNESS®

God-view	Life-view	Level		Log	Emotion	Process
Self	Is	Enlightenment	⇧	700-1000	Ineffable	Pure Consciousness
All-Being	Perfect	Peace	⇧	600	Bliss	Illumination
One	Complete	Joy	⇧	540	Serenity	Transfiguration
Loving	Benign	Love	⇧	500	Reverence	Revelation
Wise	Meaningful	Reason	⇧	400	Understanding	Abstraction
Merciful	Harmonious	Acceptance	⇧	350	Forgiveness	Transcendence
Inspiring	Hopeful	Willingness	⇧	310	Optimism	Intention
Enabling	Satisfactory	Neutrality		250	Trust	Release

Permitting	Feasible	Courage	⟺	200	Affirmation	Empowerment
Indifferent	Demanding	Pride	⇨	175	Scorn	Inflation
Vengeful	Antagonistic	Anger	⇨	150	Hate	Aggression
Denying	Disappointing	Desire	⇨	125	Craving	Enslavement
Punitive	Frightening	Fear	⇨	100	Anxiety	Withdrawal
Disdainful	Tragic	Grief	⇨	75	Regret	Despondency
Condemning	Hopeless	Apathy	⇨	50	Despair	Abdication
Vindictive	Evil	Guilt	⇨	30	Blame	Destruction
Despising	Miserable	Shame	⇨	20	Humiliation	Elimination

APPENDIX C

HOW TO CALIBRATE
THE LEVELS OF CONSCIOUSNESS

General Information

The energy field of consciousness is infinite in dimension. Specific levels correlate with human consciousness and have been calibrated from 1 to 1,000. (See Appendix B: Map of Consciousness.) These energy fields reflect and dominate human consciousness.

Everything in the universe radiates a specific frequency or minute energy field that remains in the field of consciousness permanently. Thus, every person or being that ever lived and anything about them, including any event, thought, deed, feeling, or attitude, is recorded forever and can be retrieved at any time in the present or the future.

Technique

The muscle-testing response is a simple "yes" or "not yes" (no) response to a specific stimulus. It is usually done by the subject holding out an extended arm and the tester pressing down on the wrist of the extended arm, using two fingers and light pressure. Usually the subject holds a substance to be tested over their solar plexus with the other hand. The tester says to the test subject, "Resist," and if the substance being tested is beneficial to the subject, the arm will be strong. If it is not beneficial or it has an adverse effect, the arm will go weak. The response is very quick and brief.

It is important to note that the intention, as well as both the tester and the one being tested, must calibrate over 200 in order to obtain accurate responses.

Experience from online discussion groups has shown that many students obtain inaccurate results. Further research shows that at calibration 200, there is still a 30 percent chance of error. The higher the levels of consciousness of the test team, the more accurate are the results. The best attitude is one of clinical detachment, posing a statement with the prefix statement, "In the name of the highest good, _____ calibrates as true. Over 100, Over 200," etc. The contextualization "in the highest good" increases accuracy because it transcends self-serving personal interest and motives.

For many years, the test was thought to be a local response of the body's acupuncture or immune system. Later research, however, has revealed that the response is not a local response to the body at all, but instead is a general response of consciousness itself to the energy of a substance or a statement. That which is true, beneficial, or pro-life gives a positive response that stems from the impersonal field of consciousness, which is present in everyone living. This positive response is indicated by the body's musculature going strong. There is also an associated pupillary response (the eyes dilate with falsity and constrict to truth) as well as alterations in brain function as revealed by magnetic imaging. (For convenience, the deltoid muscle is usually the one best used as an indicator muscle; however, any of the muscles of the body can be used.)

Before a question (in the form of a statement) is presented, it is necessary to qualify permission; that is, state, "I have permission to ask about what I am holding in mind" (Yes/No). Or, "This calibration serves the highest good."

If a statement is false or a substance is injurious, the muscles go weak quickly in response to the command, "Resist." This indicates the stimulus is negative, untrue, anti-life, or the answer is "no." The response is fast and brief in duration. The body will then rapidly recover and return to normal muscle tension.

There are three ways of doing the testing. The one that is used in research and also most generally used requires two people: the tester and the test subject. A quiet setting is preferred, with no background music. The test subject closes their eyes. The tester must phrase the question to be asked in the form of a statement. The statement can then be answered as "yes" or "no" by the muscle response. For instance, the *incorrect* form would be to ask, "Is this a healthy horse?" The correct form is to make the statement, "This horse is healthy," or its corollary, "This horse is sick."

After making the statement, the tester says "Resist" to the test subject who is holding the extended arm parallel to the ground. The tester presses down sharply with two fingers on the wrist of the extended arm with mild force. The test subject's arm will either stay strong, indicating a "yes," or go weak, indicating a "not yes" (no). The response is short and immediate.

A second method is the O-ring method, which can

be done alone. The thumb and middle finger of the same hand are held tightly in an O configuration, and the hooked forefinger of the opposite hand is used to try to pull them apart. There is a noticeable difference in the strength between a "yes" and a "no" response.

The third method is the simplest, yet, like the others, requires some practice. Simply lift a heavy object, such as a large dictionary or merely a couple of bricks, from a table about waist high. Hold in mind an image or true statement to be calibrated and then lift. Then, for contrast, hold in mind that which is known to be false. Note the ease of lifting when truth is held in mind and the greater effort necessary to lift the load when the issue is false (not true). The results can be verified using the other two methods.

Calibration of Specific Levels

The critical point between positive and negative, between true and false, or between that which is constructive or destructive, is at the calibrated level of 200 (see Map in Appendix B). Anything above 200, or true, makes the subject go strong; anything below 200, or false, allows the arm to go weak.

Anything past or present, including images or statements, historical events, or personages, can be tested. They need not be verbalized.

Numerical Calibration

Example: "Ramana Maharshi's teachings calibrate over 700." (Y/N). Or, "Hitler calibrated over 200." (Y/N). "When he was in his 20s." (Y/N). "His 30s." (Y/N). "His 40s." (Y/N). "At the time of his death." (Y/N).

Applications

The muscle test cannot be used to foretell the future; otherwise, there are no limits as to what can be asked. Consciousness has no limits in time or space; however, permission may be denied. All current or historical events are available for questioning. The answers are impersonal and do not depend on the belief systems of either the tester or the test subject. For example, protoplasm recoils from noxious stimuli and flesh bleeds. Those are the qualities of these test materials and are impersonal. Consciousness actually knows only truth because only truth has actual existence. It does not respond to falsehood because falsehood does not have existence in Reality. It will also not respond accurately to nonintegrous or egoistical questions.

Accurately speaking, the test response is either an "on" response or merely a "not on" response. Like the electrical switch, we say the electricity is "on," and when we use the term "off," we just mean that it is not there. In reality, there is no such thing as off-ness. This is a subtle statement but crucial to the understanding of the nature of consciousness. Consciousness is capable of recognizing only Truth. It merely fails to respond to falsehood. Similarly, a mirror reflects an image only if there is an object to reflect. If no object is present to the mirror, there is no reflected image.

To Calibrate A Level

Calibrated levels are relative to a specific reference scale. To arrive at the same figures as in the chart in Appendix A, reference must be made to that table or by a statement such as, "On a scale of human consciousness from 1 to 1,000, where 600 indicates Enlightenment, this _____ calibrates over _____ (a number)." Or, "On a scale of consciousness where 200 is the level of Truth and 500 is the level of Love, this statement calibrates over _____." (State a specific number.)

General Information

People generally want to determine truth from falsehood. Therefore, the statement has to be made very specifically. Avoid using general terms such as a good job to apply for. Good in what way? Pay scale? Working conditions? Promotional opportunities? Fairness of the boss?

Expertise

Familiarity with the test brings progressive expertise. The right questions to ask begin to spring forth and can become almost uncannily accurate. If the same tester and test subject work together for a period of time, one or both of them will develop what can become an amazing accuracy and capability of pinpointing just what specific questions to ask, even though the subject is totally unknown by either one. For instance, the tester has lost an object and begins by saying, "I left it in my office." (Answer: No.) "I left it in the car." (Answer: No.) All of a sudden, the test subject almost sees the object and says, "Ask, On the back of the bathroom door." The test subject says, "The object is hanging on the back of the bathroom door." (Answer: Yes.) In this actual case, the test subject did not even know that the tester had stopped for gas and left a jacket in the restroom of a gasoline station.

Any information can be obtained about anything anywhere in current or past time or space, depending on receiving prior permission. (Sometimes one gets a "no," perhaps for karmic or other unknown reasons.) By cross-checking, accuracy can be easily confirmed. For anyone who learns the technique, more information is available instantaneously than can be held in all the computers and libraries of the world. The possibilities are therefore obviously unlimited, and the prospects breathtaking.

Limitations

The test is accurate only if the test subjects themselves calibrate over 200 and the intention for the use of the test is integrous, calibrating over 200. The requirement is one of detached objectivity and alignment with truth rather than subjective opinion. Thus, to try to prove a point negates accuracy. Approximately 10% of the population is not able to use the kinesiologic testing technique for as yet unknown reasons. Sometimes married couples, for reasons as yet undiscovered, are unable to use each other as test subjects and may have to find a third person to be a test partner.

A suitable test subject is a person whose arm goes strong when a love object or person is held in mind, and it goes weak if that which is negative (fear, hate, guilt, etc.) is held in mind (e.g., Winston Churchill makes one go strong, and Osama bin Laden makes one go weak).

Occasionally, a suitable test subject gives paradoxical responses. This can usually be cleared by doing the thymic thump. (With a closed fist, thump three times over the upper breastbone, smile, and say "ha-ha-ha" with each thump and mentally picture someone or something that is loved.) The temporary imbalance will then clear up.

The imbalance may be the result of recently having been with negative people, listening to heavy-metal rock music, watching violent television programs, playing violent video games, etc. Negative music energy has a deleterious effect on the energy system of the body for up to one-half hour after it is turned off. Television commercials or background are also a common source of negative energy.

As previously noted, this method of discerning truth from falsehood and the calibrated levels of truth has strict requirements. Because of the limitations, calibrated levels are supplied for ready reference in *Truth vs. Falsehood*.

Explanation

The muscle-strength test is independent of personal opinion or beliefs and is an impersonal response of the field of consciousness, just as protoplasm is impersonal in its responses. This can be demonstrated by the observation that the test responses are the same whether verbalized or held silently in mind. Thus, the test subject is not influenced by the question as they do not even know what it is. To demonstrate this, do the following exercise:

The tester holds in mind an image unknown to the test subject and states, "The image I am holding in mind

is positive" (or "true," or "calibrates over 200," etc.).
Upon direction, the test subject then resists the downward pressure on the wrist. If the tester holds a positive image in mind (e.g., Abraham Lincoln, Jesus,
Mother Teresa, etc.), the test subject's arm muscle will
go strong. If the tester holds a false statement or negative image in mind (e.g., bin Laden, Hitler, etc.), the arm
will go weak. Inasmuch as the test subject does not
know what the tester has in mind, the results are not
influenced by personal beliefs.

Disqualification

Both skepticism (cal. 160) and cynicism, as well as
atheism, calibrate below 200 because they reflect negative prejudgment. In contrast, true inquiry requires an
open mind and honesty devoid of intellectual vanity.
Negative studies of the testing methodology *all* calibrate below 200 (usually at 160), as do the investigators
themselves.

That even famous professors can and do calibrate
below 200 may seem surprising to the average person.
Thus, negative studies are a consequence of negative
bias. As an example, Francis Crick's research design
that led to the discovery of the double helix pattern
of DNA calibrated at 440. His last research design,
which was intended to prove that consciousness was
just a product of neuronal activity, calibrated at only
135. (He was an atheist.)

The failure of investigators who themselves, or by
faulty research design, calibrate below 200 (usually at
160), confirms the truth of the very methodology they
claim to disprove. They should get negative results, and

so they do, which paradoxically proves the accuracy of the test to detect the difference between unbiased integrity and nonintegrity.

Any new discovery may upset the apple cart and be viewed as a threat to the status quo of prevailing belief systems. That consciousness research validates spiritual Reality is, of course, going to precipitate resistance, as it is actually a direct confrontation to the dominion of the narcissistic core of the ego itself, which is innately presumptuous and opinionated.

Below consciousness level 200, comprehension is limited by the dominance of Lower Mind, which is capable of recognizing facts but not yet able to grasp what is meant by the term truth (it confuses *res interna* with *res externa*), and that truth has physiological accompaniments that are different from falsehood. Additionally, truth is intuited as evidenced by the use of voice analysis, the study of body language, pupillary response, EEG changes in the brain, fluctuations in breathing and blood pressure, galvanic skin response, dowsing, and even the Huna technique of measuring the distance that the aura radiates from the body. Some people have a very simple technique that utilizes the standing body like a pendulum (fall forward with truth and backward with falsehood).

From a more advanced contextualization, the principles that prevail are that Truth cannot be disproved by falsehood any more than light can be disproved by darkness. The nonlinear is not subject to the limitations of the linear. Truth is a paradigm different from logic and thus is not provable, as that which is provable calibrates only in the 400s. Consciousness research methodology operates at level 600, which is at the interface of the linear and the nonlinear dimensions.

Discrepancies

Differing calibrations may be obtained over time or by different investigators for a variety of reasons:

1. Situations, people, politics, policies, and attitudes change over time.
2. People tend to use different sensory modalities when they hold something in mind, i.e., visual, sensory, auditory, or feeling. Your mother could therefore be how she looked, felt, sounded, etc., or Henry Ford could be calibrated as a father, as an industrialist, for his impact on America, his anti-Semitism, etc.
3. Accuracy increases with the level of consciousness. (The 400s and above are the most accurate.)

One can specify context and stick to a prevailing modality. The same team using the same technique will get results that are internally consistent. Expertise develops with practice. There are some people, however, who are incapable of a scientific, detached attitude and are unable to be objective, and for whom the testing method will therefore not be accurate. Dedication and intention to the truth has to be given priority over personal opinions and trying to prove them as being "right."

Note

While it was discovered that the technique does not work for people who calibrate at less than level 200, only quite recently was it further discovered that the technique does not work if the persons doing the

testing are atheists. This may be simply the consequence of the fact that atheism calibrates below level
200, and that negation of the truth or Divinity (omniscience) karmically disqualifies the negator just as hate
negates love.

REFERENCES

Abraham, R., and Shaw, C., *Dynamics: The Geometry of Behavior*, Vols. I-III. Santa Cruz, California: Aerial Press, 1984.

Amoroso, R., "Consciousness: A Radical Definition." *Toward a Scientific Basis for Consciousness; an Interdisciplinary Conference.* University of Arizona, Health Sciences Center, Tucson, Arizona, April 12-17, 1994.

Anonymous, AA *Today.* New York: Cornwall Press. 1960.

Anonymous, *A Course in Miracles.* Huntington Station, New York: Foundation for Inner Peace, Coleman-Graphics. 1975.

Anonymous, *Alcoholics Anonymous.* New York: Alcoholics Anonymous Publishing, Inc. 1955.

Anonymous, *Alcoholics Anonymous Comes of Age: A Brief History of AA.* New York: Alcoholics Anonymous Publishing, Inc. 1957.

Anonymous, *Twelve Steps and Twelve Traditions.* New York: Alcoholics Anonymous Publishing, Inc. 1953.

The Anti-Stalin Campaign and International Commission: A Selection of Documents. New York: Columbia University (Russian Institute). 1956.

Balsekar, R. S., *A Duet of One: The Ashtavatra Gita Dialogue.* Redondo Beach, California: Advaita Press. 1989.

—, *Experiencing the Teaching.* Redondo Beach, California: Advaita Press. 1988.

—, *Exploration into the Eternal.* Durham, North

Carolina: Acorn Press. 1989.

—, *The Final Truth*. Redondo Beach, California: Advaita Press. 1989.

—, *From Consciousness to Consciousness*. Redondo Beach, California: Advaita Press. 1989.

—, *Personal Interviews*. Redondo Beach, California: Advaita Press. 1987.

—, *Pointers from Nisagargadatta Maharaj*. Durham, North Carolina: Acorn Press. 1990.

Barzon, J., "The Paradoxes of Creativity." *The American Scholar*. No. 50, pp. 337-351. Summer 1989.

Bendat, J. S., and Pearson, A. G., *Measurement and Analysis of Random Data*. New York: John Wiley and Sons. 1966.

Beringa, M., "The Mind Revealed." *Science*. No. 249, pp. 156-158. August 24, 1990.

Bill W., *The Language of the Heart*. New York: Cornwall Press. 1988.

Blakney, R. B. (trans.), *Meister Eckhart*. New York: Harper & Row. 1942.

Bohm, D., *Quantum Theory*. New York: Prentice-Hall. 1980.

—, *Wholeness and the Implicate Order*. London: Routledge & Kegan Paul. 1980.

—, and Peat, F. D., *Science, Order, and Creativity*. New York: Bantam Books. 1987.

—, Hiley, B., and Kaloyerous, P. N., "An Ontological Basis for Quantum Theory." *Phys. Reports*. No. 144:6, p. 323.

Briggs, J., *Fractals: The Patterns of Chaos*. New York:

Simon & Schuster. 1993.

—, and Peat, F.D. *Looking Glass Universe*. New York: Simon & Schuster. 1984.

—, and Peat, F.D., *Turbulent Mirror: An Illustrated Guide to Chaos Theory and the Science of Wholeness*. New York: Harper & Row. 1989.

Brinkley, D., *Saved by the Light*. New York: Villard Books. 1994.

Bruner, J. S., and Posteman, L., "On the Perception of Incongruity: A Paradigm." *Journal of Personality*. No. 18, pp. 206. 1949.

Brunton, P., *A Search in Secret India*. Los Angeles: Weiser. 1984.

Butz, M., *Psychological Reports*. No. 17, pp. 827-843 and 1043-1063. 1993.

Capra, F., *The Tao of Physics: An Exploration of the Parallels Between Modern Physics and Eastern Mysticism*. New York: Bantam. 1976.

—, *The Turning Point: Science, Society, and the Rising Culture*. New York: Bantam. 1982.

Chalmers, D., "On Explaining Consciousness Scientifically: Choices and Challenges." *Toward a Scientific Basis for Consciousness; an Interdisciplinary Conference*. University of Arizona, Health Sciences Center, Tucson, Arizona, April 12-17, 1994.

Chew, G. F., "Bootstrap: A Scientific Idea." *Science*. No. 161. May 23, 1968.

—, "Hadron Bootstrap: Triumph or Frustration?" *Physics Today*. October 23, 1970.

—, "Impasse for the Elementary Particle Content." In *The Great Ideas Today*. Chicago: Encyclopedia Brittanica. 1974.

Churchill, W. S., *Blood, Sweat, and Tears*. New York: G. P. Putnam and Sons. 1941.

Combs, A., "Consciousness as a System Near the Edge of Chaos." *Toward a Scientific Basis for Consciousness; an Interdisciplinary Conference*. University of Arizona, Health Sciences Center, Tucson, Arizona, April 12-17, 1994.

Crick, F., and Koch, "The Problem of Consciousness." *Scientific American*. No. 267, pp. 152-159. September 1992.

Crusade in Europe. "1939: Marching Time." Collectors Videos.

Cuomo, M., *Lincoln on Democracy*. New York: Harper Collins. 1990.

Deikman, A. J., "The Role of Intention and Self as Determinants of Consciousness: A Functional Approach to a Spiritual Experience." *Toward a Scientific Basis for Consciousness; an Interdisciplinary Conference*. University of Arizona, Health Sciences Center, Tucson, Arizona, April 12-17, 1994.

Descartes, R., In *Great Books of the Western World*, Vol. 31. Chicago: Encyclopedia Brittanica. 1952.

Diamond, J., *Behavioral Kinesiology*. New York: Harper & Row. 1979.

—, *Your Body Doesnt Lie*. New York: Warner Books. 1979.

Dilts, R., "Strategies of Genius." *Success*. No. 39. October 26-27, 1992.

Dunn, J. (ed.), *Prior to Consciousness: Talks with Nisargadatta Maharj*. Durham, North Carolina: Acorn Press. 1985.

—, *Seeds of Consciousness*. New York: Grove Press. 1982.

Eadie, B. J., *Embraced by the Light*. Placerville, California: Gold Leaf Press. 1992.

Eccles, J., *Evolution of the Brain: Creation of the Self*. Edinburgh, Scotland: Routledge. 1989.

—, *The Human Psyche: The Gifford Lectures*. University of Edinburgh, 1977-78. Edinburgh, Scotland: Routledge. 1984.

—, (ed.), *Mind and Brain: The Many Faceted Problems*. New York: Paragon House. 1986.

—, and Robinson, D. N., *The Wonder of Being Human: Our Brain and Our Mind*. New York: Free Press. 1984.

Fedarko, K., "Escobar's Dead End." *Time*. No. 142:25, pp. 46-47. December 13, 1993.

Feigenbaum, N.J., "Universal Behavior in Nonlinear Systems." *Los Alamos Science*. No. 1, pp. 4-29. 1981.

Fischer, L., *Gandhi: His Life as a Message for the World*. New York: New American Library. 1982.

Freeman, W. J., and Skarda, C. A., "Spatial EEG Patterns: Nonlinear Dynamics and Perception." *Brain Res. Review*. No. 10, p. 147. 1985.

French, R. M. (trans.), *The Way of A Pilgrim*. New York: Seabury Press. 1965.

Galin, D., "The Structure of Subjective Experience." *Toward a Scientific Basis for Consciousness; an Interdisciplinary Conference*. University of Arizona, Health Sciences Center, Tucson, Arizona, April 12-17, 1994.

Gardner, H., *The Mind's New Science*. New York: Basic Books. 1985.

Gilbert, M., *The Complete Churchill Videos*. BBC. 1993.

Glass, L., and MacKay, M. W., "Pathological Conditions Resulting from Instabilities in Physiological Control Systems." *Ann. NY. Acad. Sci.* No. 316, p. 214. 1979.

Gleick, J., *Chaos: Making a New Science*. New York: Viking Penguin. 1987.

Godman, D. (ed.), *Be As You Are: The Teachings of Ramana Maharshi*. Boston: Arkana. 1985.

Goleman, D., et al., "The Art of Creativity." *Psychology Today*, No. 25, pp. 40-47. March/April 1992.

Goldman, A., "Philosophy of Mind: Defining Consciousness." *Toward a Scientific Basis for Consciousness; an Interdisciplinary Conference*. University of Arizona, Health Sciences Center, Tucson, Arizona, April 12-17, 1994.

Goodheart, G., *Applied Kinesiology*, 12th ed. Detroit: Privately Published. 1976.

Hardy, C., "Meaning as Interface Between Mind and Matter." *Toward a Scientific Basis for Consciousness; an Interdisciplinary Conference*. University of Arizona, Health Sciences Center, Tucson, Arizona, April 12-17, 1994.

Harman, W., "A Comparison of Three Approaches to

Reconciling Science and Consciousness." *Toward a Scientific Basis for Consciousness; an Interdisciplinary Conference*. University of Arizona, Health Sciences Center, Tucson, Arizona, April 12-17, 1994.

Hawkins, D. R., *Archival Office Visit Series*: "Stress"; "Health"; "Illness and Self-Healing"; "Handling Major Crises"; "Depression"; "Alcoholism"; "Spiritual First Aid"; "The Aging Process"; "The Map of Consciousness"; "Death and Dying"; "Pain and Suffering"; "Losing Weight"; "Worry, Fear and Anxiety"; "Drug Addiction and Alcoholism"; and "Sexuality." Lectures in video and audio. Sedona, Arizona: Institute for Spiritual Research, 1986.

—, "Consciousness and Addiction," in Kiley, L., Burton, S. (eds.), *Beyond Addictions, Beyond Boundaries*. San Mateo, California: Brookridge Institute. 1986.

—, "Expanding Love: Beauty, Silence and Joy." *Call of the Canyon*, Vol. II. Sedona, Arizona. 1983.

—, "Love, Peace and Beatitude." *Call of the Canyon*, Vol. I. Sedona, Arizona. 1982.

—, "Orthomolecular Psychiatry." *International Encyclopedia of Psychiatry, Psychoanalysis and Psychiatry*. 1979.

—, "The Prevention of Tardive Dyskinesia with High Dosage Vitamins." *Journal of Orthomolecular Medicine*. Vol. 1, No. 1. 1986.

—, and Pauling, L., *Orthomolecular Psychiatry*. San Francisco: W.H. Freeman and Company. 1973.

Heilbron, J. L., "Creativity and Big Science." *Physics*

Today. No. 45, pp. 42-47. November 1992.

Henon, J., "A Two-Dimensional Mapping with a Strange Attractor." *Com. Math Physics*. No. 50, pp. 69-77. 1976.

Hoffman, R. E., "Attractor Neuro Networks and Psychotic Disorders." *Psychiatric Annals*. No. 22:3, pp. 119-124. 1992.

Hofstadter, D. R., *Metalogical Themes: Questing for the Essence of Mind and Pattern*. Toronto, Canada: Bantam Books. 1985.

Huang Po (John Blofield, trans.), *The Zen Teaching of Huang Po: On Transmission of the Mind*. New York: Grove Press. 1958.

Insinna, E., "Synchronicity Regularities in Quantum Systems." *Toward a Scientific Basis for Consciousness; an Interdisciplinary Conference*. University of Arizona, Health Sciences Center, Tucson, Arizona, April 12-17, 1994.

James, W., *The Varieties of Religious Experience*. New York: Random House. 1929.

Josephson, M., *Edison*. New York: McGraw Hill. 1959.

Jung, C. G., *Collected Works*. Princeton, New Jersey: Princeton University Press. 1979.

—, (R. F. Hull, trans.), *Synchronicity as a Causal Connecting Principle*. Bollington Series, Vol. 20. Princeton, New Jersey: Princeton University Press. 1973.

Kaplan, B., Sedock, V., Kaplan, H., *Kaplan & Sadock's Comprehensive Textbook of Psychiatry*. Philadephia: Lippincott Williams & Wilkins. 2000.

Kelly, V. C., "Affect and Intimacy." *Psychiatric Annals*. No. 23:10 pp. 556-566. October, 1993.

Kendall, H., Kendall, F., Wadsworth, G., *Muscles: Testing and Function*. Baltimore: Williams and Wilkins. 1971.

Kosslyn, S., and Anderson, R. (eds.), *Frontiers in Cognitive Neuroscience*. Cambridge, Massachusetts: MIT Press. 1993.

Krippner, S., *Western Hemisphere Conference on Kirlian Photography*. Garden City, New York. 1974.

Kübler-Ross, E., *On Life after Death*. New York: Celestial Arts. 1991.

—, *Questions and Answers on Death and Dying*. New York: Macmillan. 1993.

Kuhn, T., *The Structure of Scientific Revolutions*. Chicago: University of Chicago Press. 1970.

Laczey, E., *Gandhi: A Man for Humanity*. New York: Hawthorne. 1972.

Lamparski, R., *Lamparski's Hidden Hollywood*. New York: Simon & Schuster. 1981.

Lamsa, G. (trans.), *Holy Bible from Ancient Eastern Manuscripts*. Philadelphia: A.J. Holmes Co. 1957.

Land, G., Jarman, B., *Breakpoint and Beyond*. New York: Harper Business. 1992.

Lash, J. P., *Roosevelt and Churchill*. New York: W. W. Norton. 1976.

Lee, T. D., *Particle Physics and Introduction to Field Theory*. Switzerland: Harwood Academic Pubs. 1981.

Li, E., and Spiegel, D., "A Neuro Network Model of

Associative Disorders." *Psychiatric Annals*. No. 22:3, pp. 144-145. 1992.

Libet, B., *Brain* 106. pp. 623-642. University of California at San Francisco Physiology Dept. 1984.

"Life's 100 Most Important Americans of the 20th Century." *Life*. No. 13:12. Fall, 1990.

"Lincoln, Abraham." In *The New Encyclopedia Brittanica*, 15th Ed. Chicago: Encyclopedia Brittanica. 1984.

Loehle, C., "A Guide to Increase Creativity in Research." *Bioscience*. No. 40, pp. 123-129. February 1990.

Lorenz, E. N., "Deterministic Nonperiodic Flow." *Journal of Atmospheric Science*. No. 20, pp. 130-141. 1963.

—, "Predictability: Does the Flap of a Butterfly's Wings Set off a Tornado in Texas?" *American Association for the Advancement of Science*. December 29, 1979.

—, "The Problem of Deducting the Climate from the Governing Equations." *Tellus*. No.16, pp. 1-11. 1964.

Lowinsky, E. A., "Musical Genius: Evolution and Origins of a Concept." *Musical Quarterly*. No. 50, pp. 321-340 and 476-495. 1964.

Maharaj, N., *I Am That*, Vols. I and II. Bombay, India: Cetana. 1973.

Maharshi, R., *Talks with Sri Ramana Maharshi*, Vols. I-III. Madras, India: Jupiter Press. 1958.

— (foreword by Carl Jung), *The Spiritual Teachings of Ramana Maharshi*. Boulder, Colorado: Shambhala. 1972.

Mandelbrot, B., *The Fractal Geometry of Nature*. New

York: W. H. Freeman and Co. 1977.

Mandell, A. J., "From Molecular Biologic Simplification to More Realistic Central Nervous System Dynamics." In Cavenar, et al. (eds.), *Psychiatry: Psychological Foundations of Clinical Psychiatry*. New York: Lippincott. 1985.

Mann, F., *The Meridians of Acupuncture*. London, England: William Heinemann Medical Books Limited. 1974.

Maslow, A. H., *The Farther Reaches of Human Nature*. New York: Viking. 1971.

McAlear, N., "On Creativity." *Omni*. No. 11, pp. 42-44. April 1989.

Mehta, V., *Mahatma Gandhi and His Apostles*. New York: Penguin Books. 1982.

"Mind's Chaotic Periods May Lead to Higher Order." *Brain/Mind Bulletin*. No. 18, p. 12.

Monroe, R., *Journeys Out of the Body*. New York: Anchor/Doubleday. 1971.

"Musical Composition." In *The New Encyclopedia Brittanica*, 15th Edition. Chicago: Encyclopedia Brittanica. 1984.

Nathanson, D. L., "About Einstein" and "Understanding Einstein." *Psychiatric Annals*. No. 23:10, pp. 543-555. October 1993.

Nome, B., *Personal Interviews*. Santa Cruz, California. 1988.

"Nonlinear Analysis Reveals Link Between Heart and Mind." *Brain/Mind Bulletin*. No. 18:12, September 1993.

Peat, F. D., *Artificial Intelligence*. New York: Baen. 1988.

—, "Time, Structure and Objectivity in Quantum Theory." *Foundation of Physics*. December 1988.

Peers, E.A. (trans.), *St. John of the Cross: Ascent of Mount Carmel*. New York: Doubleday. 1958.

Penrose, R., "Quantum Coherence and Consciousness." *Toward a Scientific Basis for Consciousness; an Interdisciplinary Conference*. University of Arizona, Health Sciences Center, Tucson, Arizona, April 12-17, 1994.

Peters, T. J., and Waterman, R. H., *In Search of Excellence*. New York: Warner Books. 1982.

Plato, *The Republic*. In *Great Books of the Western World*. Vol. 7. Chicago: Encyclopedia Brittanica, 1952.

Prigogine, I., and Stengers, I., *Order Out of Chaos: Man's New Dialogue with Nature*. Toronto, Canada: Bantam Books. 1984.

Raspberry, W., "Rap Music Shares Same Qualities as Nicotine: Dangerous, Addictive." *The Arizona Republic*. July 4, 1994.

Ray, M., and Rinzler, A. (eds.), *The New Paradigm in Business: Emerging Strategies for Leadership and Organizational Change*. New York: Tarcher/ Perigee. 1993.

Redington, D., and Reidbord, S., *Journal of Nervous and Mental Disease*. No. 180, pp. 649-665. 1992.; No. 181, pp. 428-435. 1993.

Ring, K., *Heading Toward Omega*. New York: William Morrow. 1984.

Rosband, S. N., *Chaotic Dynamics of Nonlinear Systems*. New York: John Wiley and Sons. 1990.

Rudolph, S. H., and Rudolph, L. I., *Gandhi: The Traditional Roots of Charisma*. Chicago: University of Chicago Press. 1983.

Ruelle, D., *Chaotic Evolution and Strange Attractors: The Statistical Analysis of Time Series from Deterministic Nonlinear Systems*. New York: Cambridge University Press. 1989.

—, "Strange Attractors." *Mathematical Intelligence*. No. 2, pp. 126-137. 1980.

Schaffer, W. M, and Kot, M., "Do Strange Attractors Govern Ecological Systems?" *Bioscience*. No. 35, p. 349. 1985.

Scott, A., "Hierarchical Organization in the Brain-Emergence of Consciousness." *Toward a Scientific Basis for Consciousness; an Interdisciplinary Conference*. University of Arizona, Health Sciences Center, Tucson, Arizona, April 12-17, 1994.

Sheldrake, R., *A New Science of Life*. London, England: Victoria Works. 1981.

—, Essay in *New Scientist*. No. 90, pp. 749 and 766-768. June 18, 1981.

—, "Formative Causation." Interview in *Brain/Mind Bulletin*. No. 6, p. 13. August 3, 1981.

Simonton, D. K., "What Produces Scientific Genius?" *USA Today*. No. 117, June 11, 1988.

Smale, S., *The Mathematics of Time: Essays on Dynamical Systems*. New York: Springer-Verlag. 1980.

Stewart, H. B., and Thompson, J. M., *Nonlinear Dynamics and Chaos*. New York: John Wiley & Sons. 1986.

Stone, A. M. "Implications of Affect Theory for the Practice of Cognitive Therapy." *Psychiatric Annals*. No. 23:10, pp. 577-583. 1993.

Tkacz, C., and Hawkins, D., "A Preventive Measure for Tardive Dyskinesia." *Journal of Orthomolecular Psychiatry*. Vol. 10, pp. 120-123. 1981.

Trimble, V., *Sam Walton*. New York: Dutton. 1990.

Tritton, D., "Chaos in the Swing of a Pendulum." *New Scientist*. July 24, 1986.

Tucker, R. C., *Stalin in Power*. New York: W. W. Norton. 1990.

Tuckwell, H. C., *Introduction to Theoretical Neurology: Nonlinear and Stochastic Theories*. New York: Cambridge University Press. 1988.

Varvoglis, M., "Nonlocality on a Human Scale: PSI and Consciousness Research." *Toward a Scientific Basis for Consciousness; an Interdisciplinary Conference*. University of Arizona, Health Sciences Center, Tucson, Arizona, April 12-17, 1994.

Walsh, M. (ed.), *Butler's Lives of the Saints*. New York: Harper & Row. 1985.

Walther, D., *Applied Kinesiology*. Pueblo, Colorado: Systems DC. 1976.

Weisburd, S., "Neural Nets Catch the ABCs of DNA." *Science News*. August 1, 1987.

"What is Consciousness?" Interviews with C. Koch, T. Winograd, and H. P. Moravat. In *Discover*. No. 13, pp.

95-98.

Wilber, K. (ed.), *The Holographic Paradigm and Other Paradoxes: Exploring the Leading Edge of Science.* Boston: Shambhala. 1982.

—, Engler, J., and Brown, D. P., *Transformations of Consciousness.* Boston: Shambhala. 1986.

Winfree, A., "Is It Impossible to Measure Consciousness?" *Toward a Scientific Basis for Consciousness; an Interdisciplinary Conference.* University of Arizona, Health Sciences Center, Tucson, Arizona, April 12-17, 1994.

Wing, R. L., *The Tao of Power: An Introduction to the Tao Te Ching of Lao Tsu.* Garden City, New York: Doubleday. 1986.

Wright, F. L., *Genius and the Mobocracy.* New York: Drell, Sloan, and Pierce. 1949.

Yorke, J. A., and Tien-Yien, L., "Period Three Implies Chaos." *American Math Monthly.* No. 82, pp. 985-992. 1975.

Zukav, G., *The Dancing Wu-Li Masters: An Overview of the New Physics.* New York: Bantam. 1982.

END NOTES

(See Bibliography for publication data.)

Original Foreword
1. *American Heritage Dictionary*, Houghton Mifflin, 1987.
2. See Goodheart, 1976.
3. See Diamond, 1979.
4. See Kendall, 1971.
5. Diamond, op. cit.

Original Preface
1. At this conference, for example, Richard Amoroso, Director of the Noetic Advanced Studies Institute, stated: "Consciousness is not an abstract concept but a physical reality that permeates and powers space/time which the brain mirrors. It is a multidimensional complementary continuum whose properties allow for the formation of physically testable hypotheses." "Consciousness: A Radical Definition," presented at "Toward a Scientific Basis for Consciousness: An Interdisciplinary Conference," University of Arizona Health Sciences Center, Tuscon, April 12-17, 1994.
2. See Hawkins, 1986, in Burton and Kiley.
3. Ibid.
4. Hawkins, "Consciousness and Addiction," video and audio available from Veritas Publishing.
5. Archival Office Visit Series, video and audio available from Veritas Publishing.

New Foreword
1. F. Grace, 2011. "Beyond Reason: The Certitude of the Mystic, Al-Hallaj to David R. Hawkins," *International Journal of Humanities and Social Science*, Vol. 1, No. 13 (September), 147-156.

Introduction
1. See Maharshi, 1958.
2. Polls, "Happiness is Hard to Find Anywhere in the World," *Time*, 142:11, September 13, 1993, 56.
3. See Kosslyn and Anderson, 1993.
4. See Ruelle, 1980, for a definitive discussion.
5. See Maharshi, op. cit., 118-126.

1:   Critical Advances in Knowledge
1. See Goodheart, 1976.
2. See Peat, 1988.
3. See Briggs and Peat, 1989.
4. See Walther, 1976.
5. See Lorenz, 1963.
6. See Mandelbrot, 1977.
7. Geoffrey Chew originated the Bootstrap/S-Matrix Theory and is quoted in Fritjof Capra's *The Tao of Physics* as saying that by extension, the bootstrap approach may lead to the unprecedented necessity of including the study of human consciousness explicitly in future theories of matter (1975).
8. See Bohm, 1987.
9. As Ken Wilber has pointed out, any theory of reality must include and coincide with the perennial philosophy and an ontological order of being: (1) matter; (2) biology; (3) psychology; (4) subtle/saint-

ly; (5) sage; (6) ultimate (beyond consciousness). This is discussed in Wilber's *The Holographic Paradigm*, p. 159.

10. See Maharshi, 1958.
11. See Hawkins, "Map of Consciousness," video presentation in Archival Office Series.
12. See Gleick, 1987.
13. The essentials of chaos theory are clearly explained by James Gleick in *Chaos: Making a New Science*, and by John Briggs and F. David Peat in *Turbulent Mirror*.
14. See Capra, 1975.
15. Bohm's universe is explained well by Bohm himself in an interview in *The Holographic Paradigm*, edited by Ken Wilber, 1982.
16. This state of pure awareness is Level 6 of Wilber's hierarchy, and is described in detail by Maharshi, Huang Po, and Nisargadatta Maharaj in the excellent English translations of their works cited in the Bibliography.
17. This was validated by Ramesh Balsekar who, after years of being Nisargadatta Maharaj's translator, arrived at the same state of consciousness, demonstrated during interviews (1987) and in the series of books cited in the Bibliography.
18. See Hoffman, 1992.
19. See Li and Spiegel, 1992.
20. Ibid.
21. See Hoffman, 1992.
22. See Gleick, 1987.
23. This phenomenon, called "iteration," was discussed in 1960 by Edward Lorenz in his historic

computer analysis of weather data.

24. The correlation between the work of David Bohm, Karl Pribam, Rupert Sheldrake, and Ilya Prigogine was discussed throughout the *Brain/Mind Bulletin*, Vol. IV, 1979.

25. Nobelist Sir John Eccles states that the energy of mind excites the brain to response; this is expressed in his address to the Convention of the Parapsychology Association in Utrecht, Netherlands, 1976.

2:   History and Methodology

1. See Hawkins, "Qualitative and Quantitative Analysis and Calibration of the Levels of Human Consciousness," Ph.D. dissertation, available from Veritas Publishing.

2. See Kendall, Kendall, and Wadsworth, 1971.

3. See Goodheart, 1976.

4. See Mann, 1974.

5. See Walther, 1976.

6. See Diamond, 1979.

7. See Hawkins and Pauling, editors, 1973.

8. This desynchronization was demonstrated by John Diamond at the Academy of Preventative Medicine, 1973.

9. Kinesiologic demonstrations often result in paradigm shock for people who have an investment in strict materialism. One such observer, a research psychiatrist, responded by first trying to prove that the demonstration was a fake. When he failed to do so, he walked away, saying, "Even if it's true, I don't believe it."

10. These procedures were developed over a period of several years, during regular weekly testing sessions at the Institute for Spiritual Research, Sedona, AZ, 1983-1993.
11. Hawkins, public lectures, Sedona, AZ, 1984-1989.
12. This is well documented in the field of neurolinguistic programming.
13. Diamond, lectures at the Academy of Preventative Medicine, 1978.
14. Research protocol, Institute of Spiritual Research, 1992.
15. This has been repeatedly demonstrated in public and is adequately described in Diamond's book *Your Body Doesn't Lie*.
16. The Perennial Philosophy is an extract of the spiritual truth of all religions and reflects expanding awareness on a scale progressing from matter to protoplasm, animal life, emotional responsiveness, capacity for thought, abstract thought, archetypal awareness, higher mind, saintly love and bliss, nonduality (the sage), and ultimate pure awareness. As Ken Wilber has pointed out, these strata appear universally—any theory of reality must comprehend these axioms of existence.

3: Test Results and Interpretation
1. See Eadie, p. 114.

4: Levels of Human Consciousness
1. See James, 1929.
2. Personal experience of the author.

5:   Social Distribution of Consciousness Levels
1.   The level of consciousness of mankind as a whole remained at 190 for many centuries and then suddenly jumped to its present level of 204 after the Harmonic Convergence of the late 1980s. Did the rise in consciousness bring about the Harmonic Convergence? Did the Harmonic Convergence bring about the increase in the level? Or, did a powerful, unseen "implicate order" attractor field bring about both phenomena?

6:   New Horizons in Research
1.   See Hawkins, "Consciousness and Addiction," video and audio available from Veritas Publishing.
2.   God is both transcendent (traditional religion) and immanent (the experiential truth of the mystic).
3.   *Arizona Republic*, December 20, 1993.
4.   Fedarko, "The New Kingpins," *Time*, December 13, 1993.
5.   See Josephson, 1959, p. 20.
6.   The fact-based movie that tells the whole story and its consequences was produced as "Barbarians at the Gate" and shown in 1993 on network TV.
7.   This is a traditional observation of clinicians, confirmed by the author's clinical experience over decades.

7:   Everyday Critical Point Analysis
1.   See Appendix A.
2.   See Brunton, 1984.

8: The Source of Power

1. This was a special area of research reported by Diamond in *Behavioral Kinesiology*, 1979.

2. Discussed at length in Wilbur's *Holographic Paradigm and Other Paradoxes*, 1982.

3. Bohm, D., *Brain/Mind Bulletin*, 10:10, May 27, 1985.

4. See Sheldrake, 1981.

5. Sheldrake called for a more public approach to the scientific research. In response, prizes were awarded in the U.S. ($10,000) and Britain (£250) for confirmatory tests of the hypothesis. A Morse code experiment supported the theory, and was reported by Mahlberg in *Brain/Mind Bulletin*, 10:12, July 8, 1985.

6. The mutual dependence and interpenetration of all things is observable as one leaves duality. Oneness is central to all of the major religions and spiritual systems as the ultimate reality underlying and within all forms.

7. See Land and Jarman, 1992.

9: Power Patterns in Human Attitudes

1. See Bohm, 1980.

2. See Sheldrake, 1981.

3. "Test Supports Sheldrake Theory," *Brain/Mind Bulletin*, 8:15, September 12, 1983.

10: Power in Politics

1. See Rudolph and Rudolph, 1983.

2. See Mehta, 1982.

3. See Fischer, 1982.

4. See Laczey, 1972.
5. Ibid.
6. See *Newsweek*, May 9, 1994.
7. "Crusade in Europe," *March of Time Video Series*, 1939; also Lash, 1976.
8. See Tucker, 1990.
9. This interaction between the idealism of Communism and the realities of ongoing labor wars was well presented in the PBS series *The Great Depression*, 1993.
10. Stewardship as a primary leadership role has received considerable emphasis in recent socio-political dialogue.
11. See Cuomo, *Lincoln*, 1990.
12. See Fischer, op. cit.

11: Power in the Marketplace

1. See Trimble, 1990.
2. In this classic analysis of business principles, Peters and Waterman identified the sources of power as *principles* rather than business policies and procedures, management practices, or technology.

12: Power and Sports

1. "The Big Blue" (starring Rosanna Arquette and Jean-Marc Benn), directed by Luc Besson, produced by Studio le Clare, Paris, 1985.
2. The mottoes of *Goshin-Kan* (classical Okinawan karate) are: (1) Strive for good moral character; (2) keep an honest and sincere way; (3) persevere; (4) maintain a respectful attitude; (5) restrain the

physical by spiritual attainment; and (6) cultivate and preserve life and avoid its destruction.

3. Personal karate instruction of the author by Shihan Dennis Rao, 1986.
4. Personal instruction by Master Seiyu Oyata, 1986.

13: Social Power and the Human Spirit

1. Spirit is defined in the *Living Webster Encyclopedic Dictionary* of the English Language (English Language Institute of America, Chicago, 1971) as: "Latin *spiritus*: breath, air, life essence, soul; the incorporeal principle of life, the vital principle of man, conscious being as opposed to matter; vigor, courage, aliveness; character, the divine aspect of the Trinity; the principle behind action; general meaning, active principle; dominant tendency."

2. The definition of Spirit as a concept has always presented a difficult challenge to the human intellect; a full comprehension of its significance seems beyond the capacity of the left brain (which, like a digital computer, defines how one thing differs from another). Spirit is a holistic term best grasped by the right brain (which, like an analog computer, deals with wholes and essences). The lengthy philosophical discussions that have wrestled with the idea of spirit or soul through the centuries testify to the inability of the intellect alone to deal with essence. The paradox of these philosophical debates is that any discussion at all regarding meaning utilizes essence as the very stuff of its discourse. Thus, even a discus-

sion that rejects *a priori* idea/essence/spirit does so on the presumption of the existence of truth as the basis of the argument. If there is no such thing as reality-based spirit/essence/truth, then there is no premise for any argument against their existence either, as no argument would have a reality base. In modern times, we could say that the concept of spirit refers to Bohm's implicate order, just as the concept of the corporeal refers to the explicate order.

3.   What is unique about the basic premise of the U.S. government—and the source of its power—is the concept that it derives its authority by consent of the governed, who are equal by virtue of the divinity of their Creator ("one nation under God"…).

4.   A calibrated comparison between the original spiritual foundations of the world's great religions and their subsequent formal expressions is presented in Chapter 23. There is a notably wide disparity between the two readings.

5.   The preamble to every AA meeting states: "Alcoholics Anonymous is a fellowship of men and women who share their experience, strength, and hope with each other that they may share their common problem and help others to recover from alcoholism. The only requirement for membership is a desire to stop drinking. There are no dues or fees for AA membership; we are self-supporting through our own contributions. AA is not allied with any sect, denomination, politics, organization, or institution; does not wish to engage in

any controversy, neither endorses nor opposes any causes. Our primary purpose is to stay sober and help other alcoholics to achieve sobriety." (Alcoholics Anonymous, P.O. Box 459, Grand Central Station, New York, NY, 1941, 1993.)

6. See *Twelve Steps and Twelve Traditions*, 1952.
7. See Chapter 11 in *Alcoholics Anonymous*, 1955.
8. See Bill W., 1988; *Selected Letters of C.G. Jung, 1909-1961*, 276-281.
9. Ibid., 281-286.
10. See "Bill's Story" in *Alcoholics Anonymous*, 1955, 1-17.
11. Ibid., 171-182.
12. See *Life's 100 Most Important Americans of the 20th Century*, 66.

14: Power in the Arts
1. Liner notes to *Tabula Rasa*, ECM Records, 1984.

15: Genius and the Power of Creativity
1. See Dilts, 1992.
2. Frank Lloyd Wright stated that "the Artist's perception science later verifies." (See Wright, 1949.)
3. See Goleman, 1992.
4. See Loehle, 1990.
5. See Heilbron, 1992; also Churchill, 1941.

17: Physical Health and Power
1. See Hawkins and Pauling, editors, 1973.
2. See Tkacz and Hawkins, 1981.
3. See Hawkins, 1989.
4. See Hawkins, 1991.

18: Wellness and the Disease Process
1. See Walther, 1976.
2. See Mann, 1974.
3. See Diamond, 1979.
4. See Briggs and Peat, 1989.
5. See Redington and Reidbord, 1993.
6. This is emphasized in the basic book of AA, *Alcoholics Anonymous*, 1955.
7. See Bill W., *The Language of the Heart*, 1988.
8. See *AA Comes of Age*, 1957, and *AA Today*, 1960.
9. See *Twelve Steps and Twelve Traditions*, 1953.
10. See *AA Comes of Age*, 1957.

19: The Database of Consciousness
1. See Jung, 1979.
2. Ibid. The implication of synchronicity is that two events are not causally connected in reality but are perceived so by the observer because they are meaningful. As one's consciousness advances into the high 500s, everything begins to happen by synchronicity, and the events of life unfold in perfect order and harmony with precise timing. See also Insinna, 1994.
3. See Maharshi, 1958; Maharaj, 1973; Huang Po, 1958; and Balsekar, 1987-1991.

20: The Evolution of Consciousness
1. See Eadie, 1992.
2. In an interesting coincidence, after this chapter was written, "a 75-year-old man with a tobacco-stained white beard...[who]...would not describe himself as homeless, [said] only that he was with-

out a home temporarily while 'he waited for a friend.'" This man set up an impromptu camp on public land adjacent to the highway in a community neighboring the author's. During his month's residence there, Cyrus (as he identified himself) was the center of a minor controversy. Some citizens said he was an eyesore and clamored for his removal, and the sheriff's department viewed him with suspicion and threatened to arrest him for trespassing. Others found him a harmless novelty or applauded his individualism; at least one local resident "offered him lodging, which he thought about, he said." He refused to request help from social-service organizations, "saying, 'I don't need any and don't want any,' but he did accept kindness from individuals. People came by bringing him food, particularly sandwiches, he said." (*Red Rock News*, Sedona, Arizona, November 27, 1993.) On the day of the deadline given him by sheriff's deputies, Cyrus mysteriously disappeared.
3.   See Maharaj, 1973.

21: The Study of Pure Consciousness
1.   See Descartes, "Rules for the Direction of the Mind," in *Great Books of the Western World*, v. 31, 4.
2.   See section on "Poverty" in Kaplan & Sadock's *Comprehensive Textbook of Psychiatry*, 2000, 205-287.
3.   See Maharshi, 1958; Maharaj, 1973.
4.   Ibid.
5.   See Maharaj, 1973.

6. See James, 1929.
7. Personal experience of the author.
8. See Maharaj, op. cit.; Huang Po, op. cit.; Maharshi, 1952; and Balsekar, 1987-1991.
9. See Maharaj, op. cit.; Huang Po, op. cit.; Balsekar, op. cit.
10. See *Brain/Mind Bulletin*, op. cit.
11. See Chapter 15, "Genius and the Power of Creativity."
12. See Kuhn, 1970.
13. See Kübler-Ross, 1993.
14. See Krippner, 1974.
15. Ibid.
16. See *AA Comes of Age*.
17. Bill W., 1988.
18. See Chapter 1, "Bill's Story," in *Alcoholics Anonymous*, 1952.
19. See *Twelve Steps and Twelve Traditions*.

22: Spiritual Struggle

1. See Maharshi, 1958; Huang Po, 1958; Maharaj, 1973; Balsekar, 1990.
2. See Balsekar, 1989.
3. See Walsh, 1985.
4. See Maharshi, 1958.
5. "Anguish of the Soul" is a theme throughout classic Christian literature. See Peers, 1958; Blakney, 1942; French, 1965; Walsh, 1985.
6. See Krippner, 1974.
7. See Diamond, J., *Lectures on Behavioral Kinesiology*, NY, 1972.
8. Sedona Villa of Camelback Hospital treated more

than 100 cocaine addicts a year for a five-year period (1981-1986). None of the patients who continued to listen to heavy metal rock music recovered (follow-up survey, 1986).

9. Addicts who leave 12-step programs relapse (clinical observation of the author).
10. See Maharshi, 1958.
11. See "St. Francis of Assisi," in Walsh's *Butler's Lives of the Saints*, 1985, 314-320.
12. See *A Course in Miracles*, 1975.
13. See Capra, 1976.

23: The Search for Truth

1. The fall of Christianity from a calibrated 930 to 498 must be recognized as the greatest single catastrophe in the history of Western religion. Here we can see the origin of the spiritual divorce from the actual teachings of Jesus Christ that allowed the later atrocities of the Crusades and the Inquisition. A recurrent question in speculation about the historic decline of Christianity centers around the inclusion of the relatively weak (475) Old Testament in the canon of Christian scripture. What, really, does the "eye-for-an-eye" ethic of the prophets have to do with Christ's exhortation to universal love and forgiveness? It has rightly been asked why, if Jesus came to teach the Old Testament, need he have bothered coming at all?

More to the point, as in the case of Islam, the everyday practice of Christianity is most conspicuously tainted by militant fundamentalist groups that define themselves by their hates and hawk agendas, primarily based on depriving others of their freedoms. It may well be this burden of vitriolic negativity that keeps current Christianity below the level of Love. It is interesting that these so-called Christians rarely quote Christ. Their repertory of polemic and self-justification is drawn almost entirely from the Old Testament; when they say "scripture," that is usually what they mean.

Had Christianity, in valuing moral behavior, kept exclusively to the tenets of the New Testament, one must wonder what the world would be like today.

2. Author's clinical experience.
3. Freud remained below the critical level of 500 because of his denial of man's spirituality, whereas Carl Jung, who affirmed the spiritual nature of man, calibrated at a much higher level, mid-500s.

24: Resolution

1. Socrates taught that man's purpose is to dedicate his life to the enlightenment of his soul (the light) rather than the pursuit of materialism and the senses (which leads to darkness). See Plato's *Republic*, op. cit.
2. Epistle of Paul to the Ephesians, 6:12. "For your conflict is not only with flesh and blood, but also with the angels, and with powers seen and unseen, with the rulers of the world of darkness, one with the evil spirits under the heavens." *Holy Bible*, Trans. George Lamsa, (Philadelphia: A.J.

Holmes Co., 1957).

3. This is often stated as a starting point from which to eventually arrive at a realization of our true nature, by teachers such as Nisargadatta Maharaj in *I Am That*, 1973.

GLOSSARY

Chaos Theory: The science of *process* as opposed to *state*. This theory originates in the discovery of patterns within a condition of unpredictability. The view it proposes discerns global possibilities rather than local events, and entails a topologic system using patterns and shapes to visualize the intrinsic form of a complex system which, though locally unpredictable, is globally stable. Chaos theory recognizes the capacity of a complex system to simultaneously give rise to both turbulence and coherence.

In the late 1800s, Jules-Henri Poincaré noted that Newtonian physics was mathematically accurate if the interaction studied was between two bodies only, but that the addition of a third element made Newton's equations unreliable—only approximations could be obtained. This nonlinearity implied that any system over time could, by feedback and repetition, become unpredictable. Lorenz's 1963 article, "Deterministic Nonperiodic Flow," provided a new paradigm of science, termed "Chaos Theory" by James Yorke in his famous paper, "Period Three Implies Chaos." Chaos Theory encompasses such subjects as period doubling, iteration, fractals and bifurcation, and recognizes that within finite space, there are an infinite number of dimensions. The first meeting on Chaos at the New York Academy of Science was in 1977, and in 1986, the academy had its first meeting on Chaos Theory in medicine and biology.

Context: The total field of observation predicated by a

point of view. Context includes any significant facts that qualify the meaning of a statement or event. Data is meaningless unless its context is defined. To "take out of context" is to distort the significance of a statement by failing to identify contributory accessory conditions that would qualify the inference of meaning. (This is a common trial strategy whereby an attorney tries to distort a witness's testimony by suppressing the inclusion of qualifying statements that would alter the implications of the testimony, demanding that the witness answer only "yes or no.")

Creation: A continuous process without beginning or end, through which the manifest universe of form and matter is produced by reiteration, starting from three points—all that is required to create by fractals an infinite variety of forms. (This is illustrated by the now familiar complex plane of the "Mandelbrot Set.") In Sanskrit, the three aspects of origination of all that is experienceable are called Rajas, Tamas, and Sattvas. These are symbolized by the Hindu deities Shiva, Vishnu, and Brahma. In Christianity, these are represented by the Trinity.

Duality: The world of form characterized by seeming separation of objects (reflected in conceptual dichotomies such as "this/that," "here/there," "then/now," or "you/me"). This perception of limitation is produced by the senses because of the restriction implicit in a fixed point of view. Science has finally gone beyond the artificial dichotomy of observer and observed characteristic of 17th-century Cartesian duality, and now assumes that they are one and the same. The universe has no center, but is continually expanding equally and simultaneously from every point. Bell's Theorem helped to demonstrate that this is a universe of simultaneity rather than Newtonian cause and effect over distance in an artificial time frame. Both time and space themselves are merely the measurable products of a higher implicit order.

Energy Field: In this study, a range set by parameters of the phase space of an attractor field whose pattern operates within the larger energy field of consciousness and is observable by characteristic effects in human behavior. The power of energy fields is calibrated much like voltage in an electrical system or the power of magnetic or gravitational fields.

Entrainment: A phenomenon illustrated by the principle of "mode locking." When a number of pendulum clocks are placed close together, their pendulums will eventually synchronize. In human biology this is manifested when groups of women who work or live together progressively synchronize their menstrual cycles. It is similar to the phenomenon of a tuning fork. It is because of this process that troops tend to break cadence when they cross a bridge.

Fractal: Fractal patterns are characterized by irregularity and infinite length, and strange attractors are composed of fractal curves. A classic example is the attempt to determine the length of the coastline of Britain. If one adds lengths using smaller and smaller scales of measurement, it turns out to be infinitely long. Fractal implies an infinite length in a finite area.

Hologram: A three-dimensional projection into space of the image of an object, created by projecting laser light so that half of the beam is directed to the object and then onto a photographic plate, which receives the other half of the beam directly. This creates an interference pattern on the plate so that a laser beam projected through the plate recreates the image of the object in three dimensions. It is of interest that every fragment of the photographic plate is capable of reproducing the entire image of the whole. In a holographic universe, everything is connected to everything else.

Iteration: Repetition. Nonlinear iteration is present in innumerable systems. Because of this repetition, a very slight change in the initial condition will eventually produce a pattern dissimilar from the original. In a growth equation, the output of the prior iteration becomes the input for the next series. For example, if a computer calculates to sixteen decimal places, the last digit is the rounding off of the seventeenth. This infinitesimal error, magnified through many iterations results in substantial distortion of the original data and makes prediction impossible. (Thus, a slight change in a repetitious thought pattern can bring about major effects.)

Left-brain: Referring to thought sequenced in the linear style, which is commonly described as "logic" or "reason." Processing of data in a sequence A→B→C. Analogous to a digital computer.

Linear: Following a logical progression in the manner of Newtonian physics and, therefore, solvable by traditional mathematics through the use of differential equations.

M-Fields: Morphogenetic fields, analogous to attractor patterns. In the hypothesis presented by Rupert Sheldrake, morphogenetic fields are part of the theory of formative causation, that energy fields of form evolve and reinforce each other.

Neural Network: The interlocking patterns of interacting neurons within the nervous system.

Neurotransmitters: Brain chemicals (hormones, etc.) that regulate neuronal transmission throughout the nervous system. Very slight chemical changes can result in major subjective and objective alterations in emotion, thought, or behavior. This is the prime area of current research in psychiatry.

Non-duality: Historically, all observers who have reached a consciousness level over 600 have described the reality now suggested by advanced scientific theory. When the limitation of a fixed locus of perception is transcended, there is no longer an illusion of separation, nor of space and time as we know them. All things exist simultaneously in the unmanifest, enfolded, implicit universe, expressing itself as the manifest, unfolded, explicit perception of form. These forms in reality have no intrinsic, independent existence but are the product of perception (that is, man is merely experiencing the content of his own mind). On the level of non-duality, there is observing but no observer, as subject and object are one. You-and-I becomes the One Self experiencing all as divine. At level 700, it can only be said that "All Is;" the state is one of Being-ness; all is consciousness, which is infinite, which is God and which has no parts or a beginning or end. The physical body is a manifestation of the One Self which, in experiencing this dimension, had temporarily forgotten its reality, thus permitting the illusion of a three-dimensional world. The body is merely a means of communication; to identify one's self with the body as "I" is the fate of the unenlightened, who then erroneously deduce that they are mortal and subject to death. Death itself is an illusion, based on the false identification with the body as "I." In non-duality, consciousness experiences itself as both manifest and unmanifest, yet there is no experiencer. In this Reality, the only thing that has a beginning and an end is the act of perception itself. In the illusory world, we are like the fool who believes that things come into existence when he opens his eyes and cease to exist when he closes them.

Nonlinear: Unpredictably irregular in time, "noisy," nonperiodic, random, and stochastic. Illustrated by mathematical series such as formulized stochastic evolution equations of the form $dx(t)dt=F(xt)+w(t)$

where $w(t)$ is the noise term of the stochastic process. The term also describes the mathematics of chaotic signals, including the statistical analysis of time series for deterministic nonlinear systems. Nonlinear means diffuse or chaotic; not in accordance with probabilistic logical theory or mathematics; not solvable by differential equations. This is the subject of the science of Chaos Theory, which has given rise to a whole new non-Newtonian mathematics.

Oxymoronic: An expression of complexity or ambiguity in deceptively simple, apparently contradictory terms. The resolution of contradiction by juxtaposition and contrast, as in "cold fire" or "wise fool." Oxymoronic styles reflect the essence of paradox, and paradox itself arises from the contrast between different levels of abstraction, occasioned by the presentation of concepts from different contexts and points of view.

Paradigm: The dimensions of a context or field as limited by parameters that inherently predict one's perception of reality. A paradigm, generally, is a definition of one's perception of reality according to its limitations.

Phase space: A map that affords the condensation of time-space data into a pattern in multiple dimensions. A Poincaré map is the graphic depiction of a slice through a multidimensional pattern that demonstrates the underlying attractor.

Right-brain: Generally meaning "holistic"; enabling such functions as evaluation, intuition, and comprehension of significance, meaning, and inference. Nonlinear; operating from patterns and relationships rather than through the logical sequences of Newtonian causality.

The right brain is assumed to deal with wholes rather than parts. Like an analog computer, it deals with processes and is generally capable of operating without the necessity of time reference. Right-brain perception detects essence within a complex field of data that might not otherwise lend itself to meaningful cognitive analysis—such general phenomena as "falling in love" or creativity. (The terms "left-brain" and "right-brain" originated in reference to different styles of perception that were once thought to be localized to certain cerebral areas, but as Karl Pribam has shown, the brain acts holographically rather than by precise anatomic localization.)

Scientific: The method of inquiry into nature specifically designed to derive predictable laws of physical properties. Modern scientific theory began in the sixteenth century with René Descartes's *Discourse on Method*, followed by Francis Bacon's *Inductive Inquiry*, and Isaac Newton's *Principia*. John Locke first used the term "scientific" and proposed that certainty about the interaction of physical events was based on data arrived at by physical sensation. These concepts resulted in a model of a mechanical, predictive universe, but this view was upset by a modern quantum theory, which states that at the subatomic level, the laws of chance replace deterministic laws.

History has noted that science does not advance by an extension of established theories, but instead takes leaps by a shift of paradigm. The inference is that science is merely a reflection of a point of view, and there is no real separation between observer and observed. Relativity theory further states that matter equals energy, depending on one's point of reference. David Bohm's later *Holographic Model* predicates an explicit order based on an implicit order. Form becomes the consequence of inference, space and time are non-localized, and there is no "here" or "there" (the non-locality of quantum wholeness). The universe thus described contains an infinite number of dimensions and higher-dimension realities.

Stochastic: Random, unpredictable, nonlinear, erratic, "noisy," chaotic.

Strange Attractor: A term coined by David Ruelle and Floris Takens in 1971, in a theory that stated that three independent motions are all that is necessary to produce the entire complexity of nonlinear patterns of the universe. A strange attractor is a pattern within a phase space. The pattern is traced by the dynamic points in time of a dynamic system. The central point of an attractor field is analogous to the center of an orbit. Attractors are fractal and therefore of infinite length. The graphics of attractors are depicted by taking a cross section of a so-called Poincaré map. The topographical shaping of phase space creates an attractor such as a torus, like a folded donut.

Universe: There may be seen to be an infinite number of dimensions to our universe. The familiar three-dimensional universe of conventional consensus is only one, and is merely an illusion created by our senses. The space between planetary bodies is not empty, but filled with a sea of energy; the potential energy in one square inch can be said to be as great as that of the whole mass of the physical universe. David Bohm has proposed the model of enfolded/unfolded states of being, with an explicit order and an implicit order of reality, comparable to the manifest/unmanifest states of reality that have been described for centuries by those who have achieved enlightenment and experienced non-duality.

In the causality model:

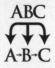

the A→B→C is the unfolded, explicit, manifest, discernible universe of form. The ABC is the enfolded, implicit, unmanifest potential beyond which is the formless, infinite matrix of both form and non-form, which is omnipotent, omniscient, and omnipresent.

ABOUT THE AUTHOR

Biographical and Autobiographical Notes

Dr. Hawkins is an internationally known spiritual teacher, author, and speaker on the subject of advanced spiritual states, consciousness research, and the Realization of the Presence of God as Self.

His published works, as well as recorded lectures, have been widely recognized as unique in that a very advanced state of spiritual awareness occurred in an individual with a scientific and clinical background who was later able to verbalize and explain the unusual phenomenon in a manner that is clear and comprehensible.

The transition from the normal ego-state of mind to its elimination by the Presence is described in the trilogy *Power vs. Force* (1995) which won praise even from Mother Teresa, *The Eye of the I* (2001), and *I: Reality and Subjectivity* (2003), which have been translated into the major languages of the world. *Truth vs. Falsehood: How to Tell the Difference* (2005), *Transcending the Levels of Consciousness* (2006), *Discovery of the Presence of God: Devotional Nonduality* (2007), and *Reality, Spirituality and Modern Man* (2008) continue the exploration of the ego's expressions and inherent limitations and how to transcend them.

The trilogy was preceded by research on the Nature of Consciousness and published as the doctoral dissertation, *Qualitative and Quantitative Analysis and Calibration of the Levels of Human Consciousness* (1995), which correlated the seemingly disparate domains of science and spirituality. This was accomplished by the major discovery of a technique that, for the first time in human history, demonstrated a means to discern truth from falsehood.

The importance of the initial work was given recognition by its very favorable and extensive review in *Brain/Mind Bulletin* and at later presentations such as the International Conference on Science and Consciousness. Many presentations were given to a variety of organizations, spiritual conferences, church groups, nuns, and monks, both nationally and in foreign countries, including the Oxford Forum in England. In the Far East, Dr. Hawkins is a recognized "Teacher of the Way to Enlightenment" ("Tae Ryoung Sun Kak Dosa"). In response to his observation that much spiritual truth has been misunderstood over the ages due to lack of explanation, Dr. Hawkins has presented monthly seminars that provide detailed explanations which are too lengthy to describe in book format. Recordings are available that end with questions and answers, thus providing additional clarification.

The overall design of this lifetime work is to recontextualize the human experience in terms of the evolution of consciousness and to integrate a comprehension of both mind and spirit as expressions of the innate Divinity that is the substrate and ongoing source of life and Existence. This dedication is signified by the statement *"Gloria in Excelsis Deo!"* with which his published works begin and end.

Biographic Summary

Dr. Hawkins has practiced psychiatry since 1952 and is a life member of the American Psychiatric Association and numerous other professional organizations. His national television appearance schedule has included *The McNeil/Leher News Hour, The Barbara Walters Show, The Today Show*, science documentaries, and many others. He was also interviewed by Oprah Winfrey.

Dr. Hawkins is the author of numerous scientific and spiritual publications, books, CDs, DVDs, and lecture series. He co-edited the landmark book, *Orthomolecular Psychiatry*, with Nobelist Linus Pauling. Dr. Hawkins was a consultant for many years to Episcopal and Catholic Dioceses, monastic orders, and other religious orders.

Dr. Hawkins has lectured widely, with appearances at Westminster Abbey, the Universities of Argentina, Notre Dame, and Michigan; Fordham University and Harvard University; and the Oxford Forum in England. He gave the annual Landsberg Lecture at the University of California Medical School at San Francisco. He is also a consultant to foreign governments on international diplomacy and was instrumental in resolving long-standing conflicts that were major threats to world peace.

In recognition of his contributions to humanity, in 1995, Dr. Hawkins became a knight of the Sovereign Order of the Hospitaliers of St. John of Jerusalem, which was founded in 1077.

Autobiographic Note

While the truths reported in this book were scientifically derived and objectively organized, like all truths, they were first experienced personally. A lifelong sequence of intense states of awareness beginning at a young age first inspired and then gave direction to the process of subjective realization that has finally taken form in this series of books.

At age three, there occurred a sudden full consciousness of existence, a nonverbal but complete understanding of the meaning of "I Am," followed immediately by the frightening realization that "I" might not have come into existence at all. This was an instant awakening from oblivion into a conscious awareness, and in that moment, the personal self was born and the duality of "Is" and "Is Not" entered my subjective awareness.

Throughout childhood and early adolescence, the paradox of existence and the question of the reality of the self remained a repeated concern. The personal self would sometimes begin slipping back into a greater impersonal Self, and the initial fear of non-existence—the fundamental fear of nothingness—would recur.

In 1939, as a paperboy with a seventeen-mile bicycle route in rural Wisconsin, on a dark winter's night I was caught miles from home in a twenty-below-zero blizzard. The bicycle fell over on the ice and the fierce wind ripped the newspapers out of the handlebar basket, blowing them across the ice-covered, snowy field. There were tears of frustration and exhaustion and my clothes were frozen stiff. To get out of the wind, I broke through the icy crust of a high snow bank, dug out a space, and crawled into it. Soon the shivering stopped and there was a delicious warmth, and then a state of peace beyond all description. This was accompanied by a suffusion of light and a presence of infinite love that had no beginning and no end and was undifferentiated from my own essence. The physical body and surroundings faded as my awareness was fused with this all-present, illuminated state. The mind grew silent; all thought stopped. An infinite Presence was all that was or could be, beyond all time or description.

After that timelessness, there was suddenly an awareness of someone shaking my knee; then my father's anxious face appeared. There was great reluctance to return to the body and all that that entailed, but because of my father's love and anguish, the Spirit nurtured and reactivated the body. There was compassion for his fear of death, although, at the same time, the concept of death seemed absurd.

This subjective experience was not discussed with anyone since there was no context available from which to describe it. It was not common to hear of spiritual experiences other than those reported in the lives of the saints. But after this experience, the accepted reality of the world began to seem only provisional; traditional religious teachings lost significance and, paradoxically, I became an agnostic. Compared to the light of Divinity that had illuminated all existence, the god of traditional religion shone dully indeed; thus spirituality replaced religion.

During World War II, hazardous duty on a

minesweeper often brought close brushes with death, but there was no fear of it. It was as though death had lost its authenticity. After the war, fascinated by the complexities of the mind and wanting to study psychiatry, I worked my way through medical school. My training psychoanalyst, a professor at Columbia University, was also an agnostic; we both took a dim view of religion. The analysis went well, as did my career, and success followed.

I did not, however, settle quietly into professional life. I fell ill with a progressive, fatal illness that did not respond to any treatments available. By age 38, I was *in extremis* and knew I was about to die. I didn't care about the body, but my spirit was in a state of extreme anguish and despair. As the final moment approached, the thought flashed through my mind, "What if there is a God?" So I called out in prayer, "If there is a God, I ask him to help me now." I surrendered to whatever God there might be and went into oblivion. When I awoke, a transformation of such enormity had taken place that I was struck dumb with awe.

The person I had been no longer existed. There was no personal self or ego, only an Infinite Presence of such unlimited power that it was all that was. This Presence had replaced what had been "me," and the body and its actions were controlled solely by the Infinite Will of the Presence. The world was illuminated by the clarity of an Infinite Oneness that expressed itself as all things revealed in their infinite beauty and perfection.

As life went on, this stillness persisted. There was no personal will; the physical body went about its business under the direction of the infinitely powerful but exquisitely gentle Will of the Presence. In that state, there was no need to think about anything. All truth was self-evident and no conceptualization was necessary or even possible. At the same time, the physical nervous system felt extremely overtaxed, as though it were carrying far more energy than its circuits had been designed for.

It was not possible to function effectively in the world. All ordinary motivations had disappeared, along with all fear and anxiety. There was nothing to seek, as all was perfect. Fame, success, and money were meaningless. Friends urged the pragmatic return to clinical practice, but there was no ordinary motivation to do so.

There was now the ability to perceive the reality that underlay personalities: the origin of emotional sickness lay in people's belief that they *were* their personalities. And so, as though of its own, a clinical practice resumed and eventually became huge.

People came from all over the United States. The practice had two thousand outpatients, which required more than fifty therapists and other employees, a suite of twenty-five offices, and research and electroencephalic laboratories. There were a thousand new patients a year. In addition, there were appearances on radio and network television shows, as previously mentioned. In 1973, the clinical research was documented in a traditional format in the book, *Orthomolecular Psychiatry*. This work was ten years ahead of its time and created something of a stir.

The overall condition of the nervous system improved slowly, and then another phenomenon commenced. There was a sweet, delicious band of energy continuously flowing up the spine and into the brain where it created an intense sensation of continuous pleasure. Everything in life happened by synchronicity, evolving in perfect harmony; the miraculous was commonplace. The origin of what the world would call miracles was the Presence, not the personal self. What remained of the personal "me" was only a witness to these phenomena. The greater "I," deeper than my former self or thoughts, determined all that happened.

The states that were present had been reported by others throughout history and led to the investigation of spiritual teachings, including those of the Buddha, enlightened sages, Huang Po, and more recent teachers such as Ramana Maharshi and Nisargadatta Maharaj. It was thus confirmed that these experiences were not unique. The *Bhagavad-Gita* now made complete sense. At times, the same spiritual ecstasy reported by Sri Ramakrishna and the Christian saints occurred.

Everything and everyone in the world was luminous and exquisitely beautiful. All living beings became Radiant and expressed this Radiance in stillness and splendor. It was apparent that all mankind is actually motivated by inner love but has simply become unaware; most lives are lived as though by sleepers unawakened to the awareness of who they really are. People around me looked as though they were asleep and were incredibly beautiful. It was like being in love with everyone.

It was necessary to stop the habitual practice of meditating for an hour in the morning and then again before dinner because it would intensify the bliss to such an extent that it was not possible to function. An experience similar to the one that had occurred in the snow bank as a boy would recur, and it became increasingly difficult to leave that state and return to the world. The incredible beauty of all things shone forth in all their perfection, and where the world saw ugliness, there was only timeless beauty. This spiritual love suffused all perception, and all boundaries between here and there, or then and now, or separation disappeared.

During the years spent in inner silence, the strength of the Presence grew. Life was no longer personal; a personal will no longer existed. The personal "I" had become an instrument of the Infinite Presence and went about and did as it was willed. People felt an extraordinary peace in the aura of that Presence. Seekers sought answers but as there was no longer any such individual as David, they were actually finessing answers from their own Self, which was not different from mine. From each person the same Self shone forth from their eyes.

The miraculous happened, beyond ordinary comprehension. Many chronic maladies from which the body had suffered for years disappeared; eyesight spontaneously normalized, and there was no longer a need for the lifetime bifocals.

Occasionally, an exquisitely blissful energy, an Infinite Love, would suddenly begin to radiate from the heart toward the scene of some calamity. Once, while driving on a highway, this exquisite energy began to beam out of the chest. As the car rounded a bend, there was an auto accident; the wheels of the over-

turned car were still spinning. The energy passed with
great intensity into the occupants of the car and then
stopped of its own accord. Another time, while I was
walking on the streets of a strange city, the energy
started to flow down the block ahead and arrived at
the scene of an incipient gang fight. The combatants
fell back and began to laugh, and again, the energy
stopped.

Profound changes of perception came without
warning in improbable circumstances. While dining
alone at Rothmann's on Long Island, the Presence suddenly intensified until every thing and every person,
which had appeared as separate in ordinary perception, melted into a timeless universality and oneness. In
the motionless Silence, it became obvious that there
are no "events" or "things" and that nothing actually
"happens" because past, present, and future are merely
artifacts of perception, as is the illusion of a separate "I"
being subject to birth and death. As the limited, false
self dissolved into the universal Self of its true origin,
there was an ineffable sense of having returned home
to a state of absolute peace and relief from all suffering.
It is only the illusion of individuality that is the origin
of all suffering. When one realizes that one is the universe, complete and at one with All That Is, forever
without end, then no further suffering is possible.

Patients came from every country in the world,
and some were the most hopeless of the hopeless.
Grotesque, writhing, wrapped in wet sheets for transport from far-away hospitals they came, hoping for
treatment for advanced psychoses and grave, incurable mental disorders. Some were catatonic; many

had been mute for years. But in each patient, beneath the crippled appearance, there was the shining essence of love and beauty, perhaps so obscured to ordinary vision that he or she had become totally unloved in this world.

One day a mute catatonic was brought into the hospital in a straitjacket. She had a severe neurological disorder and was unable to stand. Squirming on the floor, she went into spasms and her eyes rolled back in her head. Her hair was matted; she had torn all her clothes and uttered guttural sounds. Her family was fairly wealthy; as a result, over the years she had been seen by innumerable physicians and famous specialists from all over the world. Every treatment had been tried on her and she had been given up as hopeless by the medical profession.

A short, nonverbal question arose: "What do you want done with her, God?" Then came the realization that she just needed to be loved, that was all. Her inner self shone through her eyes and the Self connected with that loving essence. In that second, she was healed by her own recognition of who she really was; what happened to her mind or body did not matter to her any longer.

This, in essence, occurred with countless patients. Some recovered in the eyes of the world and some did not, but whether a clinical recovery ensued did not matter any longer to the patients. Their inner agony was over. As they felt loved and at peace within, their pain stopped. This phenomenon can only be explained by saying that the Compassion of the Presence recontextualized each patient's reality so

that he or she experienced healing on a level that transcended the world and its appearances. The inner
peace of the Self encompassed us beyond time and
identity.

It was clear that all pain and suffering arises solely
from the ego and not from God. This truth was silently
communicated to the minds of the patients. This was
the mental block in another mute catatonic who had
not spoken in many years. The Self said to him through
mind, "You're blaming God for what your ego has done
to you." He jumped off the floor and began to speak,
much to the shock of the nurse who witnessed the
incident.

The work became increasingly taxing and eventually
overwhelming. Patients were backed up, waiting for
beds to open, although the hospital had built an extra
ward to house them. There was an enormous frustration in that the human suffering could be countered in
only one patient at a time. It was like bailing out the
sea. It seemed that there must be some other way to
address the causes of the common malaise, the endless
stream of spiritual distress and human suffering.

This led to the study of the physiological response
(muscle testing) to various stimuli, which revealed an
amazing discovery. It was the "wormhole" between two
universes—the physical world and the world of the
mind and spirit—an interface between dimensions. In
a world full of sleepers lost from their source, here was
a tool to recover, and demonstrate for all to see, that
lost connection with the higher reality. This led to the
testing of every substance, thought, and concept that
could be brought to mind. The endeavor was aided by

my students and research assistants. Then a major discovery was made: whereas all subjects went weak from negative stimuli, such as fluorescent lights, pesticides, and artificial sweeteners, students of spiritual disciplines who had advanced their levels of awareness did not go weak as did ordinary people. Something important and decisive had shifted in their consciousness. It apparently occurred as they realized they were not at the mercy of the world but rather affected only by what their minds believed. Perhaps the very process of progress toward enlightenment could be shown to increase man's ability to resist the vicissitudes of existence, including illness.

The Self had the capacity to change things in the world by merely envisioning them; Love changed the world each time it replaced non-love. The entire scheme of civilization could be profoundly altered by focusing this power of love at a very specific point. Whenever this happened, history bifurcated down new roads.

It now appeared that these crucial insights could not only be communicated with the world but also visibly and irrefutably demonstrated. It seemed that the great tragedy of human life had always been that the psyche is so easily deceived; discord and strife have been the inevitable consequence of mankind's inability to distinguish the false from the true. But here was an answer to this fundamental dilemma, a way to recontextualize the nature of consciousness itself and make explicable that which otherwise could only be inferred.

It was time to leave life in New York, with its city

apartment and home on Long Island, for something more important. It was necessary to perfect myself as an instrument. This necessitated leaving that world and everything in it, replacing it with a reclusive life in a small town where the next seven years were spent in meditation and study.

Overpowering states of bliss returned unsought, and eventually, there was the need to learn how to be in the Divine Presence and still function in the world. The mind had lost track of what was happening in the world at large. In order to do research and writing, it was necessary to stop all spiritual practice and focus on the world of form. Reading the newspaper and watching television helped to catch up on the story of who was who, the major events, and the nature of the current social dialogue.

Exceptional subjective experiences of truth, which are the province of the mystic who affects all mankind by sending forth spiritual energy into the collective consciousness, are not understandable by the majority of mankind and are therefore of limited meaning except to other spiritual seekers. This led to an effort to be ordinary, because just being ordinary in itself is an expression of Divinity; the truth of one's real self can be discovered through the pathway of everyday life. To live with care and kindness is all that is necessary. The rest reveals itself in due time. The commonplace and God are not distinct.

And so, after a long circular journey of the spirit, there was a return to the most important work, which was to try to bring the Presence at least a little closer to the grasp of as many fellow beings as possible.

The Presence is silent and conveys a state of peace that is the space in which and by which all is and has its existence and experience. It is infinitely gentle and yet like a rock. With it, all fear disappears. Spiritual joy occurs on a quiet level of inexplicable ecstasy. Because the experience of time stops, there is no apprehension or regret, no pain or anticipation; the source of joy is unending and ever present. With no beginning or ending, there is no loss or grief or desire. Nothing needs to be done; everything is already perfect and complete.

When time stops, all problems disappear; they are merely artifacts of a point of perception. As the Presence prevails, there is no further identification with the body or the mind. When the mind grows silent, the thought "I Am" also disappears, and Pure Awareness shines forth to illuminate what one is, was, and always will be, beyond all worlds and all universes, beyond time, and therefore without beginning or end.

People wonder, "How does one reach this state of awareness," but few follow the steps because they are so simple. First, the desire to reach that state was intense. Then began the discipline to act with constant and universal forgiveness and gentleness, without exception. One has to be compassionate towards everything, including one's own self and thoughts. Next came a willingness to hold desires in abeyance and surrender personal will at every moment. As each thought, feeling, desire, or deed was surrendered to God, the mind became progressively silent. At first, it released whole stories and paragraphs, then ideas and concepts. As one lets go of wanting to own these thoughts, they no longer reach such elaboration and begin to fragment while only half formed. Finally, it was possible to turn over the energy behind thought itself before it even became thought.

The task of constant and unrelenting fixity of focus, allowing not even a moment of distraction from meditation, continued while doing ordinary activities. At first, this seemed very difficult, but as time went on, it became habitual, automatic, requiring less and less effort, and finally, it was effortless. The process is like a rocket leaving the earth. At first, it requires enormous power, then less and less as it leaves the earth's gravitational field, and finally, it moves through space under its own momentum.

Suddenly, without warning, a shift in awareness occurred and the Presence was there, unmistakable and all encompassing. There were a few moments of apprehension as the self died, and then the absoluteness of the Presence inspired a flash of awe. This breakthrough was spectacular, more intense than anything before. It has no counterpart in ordinary experience. The profound shock was cushioned by the love that is with the Presence. Without the support and protection of that love, one would be annihilated.

There followed a moment of terror as the ego clung to its existence, fearing it would become nothingness. Instead, as it died, it was replaced by the Self as Everythingness, the All in which everything is known and obvious in its perfect expression of its own essence. With nonlocality came the awareness that one is all that ever was or can be. One is total and complete, beyond all identities, beyond all gender, beyond even humanness itself. One need never again fear suffering and death.

What happens to the body from this point is immaterial. At certain levels of spiritual awareness, ailments of the body heal or spontaneously disappear. But in the absolute state, such considerations are irrelevant. The body will run its predicted course and then return from whence it came. It is a matter of no importance; one is unaffected. The body appears as an "it" rather than as a "me," as another object, like the furniture in a room. It may seem comical that people still address the body as though it were the individual "you," but there is no way to explain this state of awareness to the unaware. It is best to just go on about one's business and allow Providence to handle the social adjustments. However, as one reaches bliss, it is very difficult to conceal that state of intense ecstasy. The world may be dazzled, and people may come from far and wide to be in the accompanying aura. Spiritual seekers and the spiritually curious may be attracted, as may be the very ill who are seeking miracles. One may become a magnet and a source of joy to them. Commonly, there is a desire at this point to share this state with others and to use it for the benefit of all.

The ecstasy that accompanies this condition is not initially absolutely stable; there are also moments of great agony. The most intense occur when the state fluctuates and suddenly ceases for no apparent reason. These times bring on periods of intense despair and a fear that one has been forsaken by the Presence. These falls make the path arduous, and to surmount these reversals requires great will. It finally becomes obvious that one must transcend this level or constantly suffer excruciating "descents from grace." The glory of ecstasy, then, has to be relinquished as one enters upon the arduous task of transcending duality until one is beyond all opposites and their conflicting pulls. But while it is one thing to happily give up the iron chains of the ego, it is quite another to abandon the golden chains of ecstatic joy. It feels as though one is giving up God, and a new level of fear arises, never before anticipated. This is the final terror of absolute aloneness.

To the ego, the fear of nonexistence was formidable, and it drew back from it repeatedly as it seemed to approach. The purpose of the agonies and the dark nights of the soul then became apparent. They are so intolerable that their exquisite pain spurs one on to the extreme effort required to surmount them. When vacillation between heaven and hell becomes unendurable, the desire for existence itself has to be surrendered. Only once this is done may one finally move beyond the duality of Allness versus nothingness, beyond existence versus nonexistence. This culmination of the inner work is the most difficult phase, the ultimate watershed, where one is starkly aware that the illusion of existence one transcends is irrevocable. There is no returning from this step, and this specter of irreversibility makes this last barrier appear to be the most formidable choice of all.

But, in fact, in this final apocalypse of the self, the dissolution of the sole remaining duality of existence versus nonexistence—identity itself—dissolves in Universal Divinity, and no individual consciousness is left to choose. The last step, then, is taken by God.

—*David R. Hawkins*

INDEX

Hay House Titles of Related Interest

We hope you enjoyed this Hay House book. If you'd like to receive our online catalog featuring additional information on Hay House books and products, or if you'd like to find out more about the Hay Foundation, please contact:

Hay House, Inc., P.O. Box 5100, Carlsbad, CA 92018-5100
(760) 431-7695 or (800) 654-5126
(760) 431-6948 (fax) or (800) 650-5115 (fax)
www.hayhouse.com® • www.hayfoundation.org

————

Published in Australia by: Hay House Australia Pty. Ltd.,
18/36 Ralph St., Alexandria NSW 2015
Phone: 612-9669-4299 • *Fax:* 612-9669-4144
www.hayhouse.com.au

Published in the United Kingdom by: Hay House UK, Ltd.,
The Sixth Floor, Watson House, 54 Baker Street, London W1U 7BU
Phone: +44 (0)20 3927 7290 • *Fax:* +44 (0)20 3927 7291
www.hayhouse.co.uk

Published in India by: Hay House Publishers India,
Muskaan Complex, Plot No. 3, B-2, Vasant Kunj, New Delhi 110 070
Phone: 91-11-4176-1620 • *Fax:* 91-11-4176-1630
www.hayhouse.co.in

————

Access New Knowledge.
Anytime. Anywhere.

Learn and evolve at your own pace
with the world's leading experts.

www.hayhouseU.com

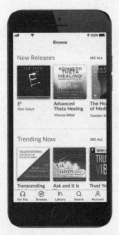